Helicobacter pylori Infection - An Up to Date on the Pathogenic Mechanisms, Diagnosis and Clinical Management

Edited by Daniela Cornelia Lazăr

Published in London, United Kingdom

Helicobacter pylori Infection - An Up to Date on the Pathogenic Mechanisms, Diagnosis and Clinical Management
http://dx.doi.org/10.5772/intechopen.104289
Edited by Daniela Cornelia Lazăr

Contributors
Alexey A. Krasnov, Amar P. Garg, Asma'a Ali Hejaze, Chenxiao Hu, Daniela Cornelia Lazăr, Helge L. Waldum, Mihaela-Flavia Avram, Natalia V. Baryshnikova, Natalie Tai, Neha Bisht, Saleh Nazmy Mwafy, Sampson Weytey, Sergey V. Petlenko, Sorin Olariu, Ting Lei, Vera A. Apryatina, Wesam Mohammad Afana, Xiujing Feng, Yan Li, Yulia A. Fominykh, Yun Lu, Yury P. Uspenskiy, Zhi Huang

First published in London, United Kingdom, 2024 by IntechOpen
IntechOpen is the global imprint of INTECHOPEN LIMITED, registered in England and Wales, registration number: 11086078, 167-169 Great Portland Street, London, W1W 5PF, United Kingdom

British Library Cataloguing-in-Publication Data
A catalogue record for this book is available from the British Library

Additional hard and PDF copies can be obtained from orders@intechopen.com

Helicobacter pylori Infection - An Up to Date on the Pathogenic Mechanisms, Diagnosis and Clinical Management
Edited by Daniela Cornelia Lazăr
p. cm.
Print ISBN 978-1-83768-170-9
Online ISBN 978-1-83768-171-6
eBook (PDF) ISBN 978-1-83768-172-3

For EU product safety concerns:
IN TECH d.o.o., Prolaz Marije Krucifikse Kozulić 3, 51000 Rijeka, Croatia,
info@intechopen.com or visit our website at intechopen.com.

Meet the editor

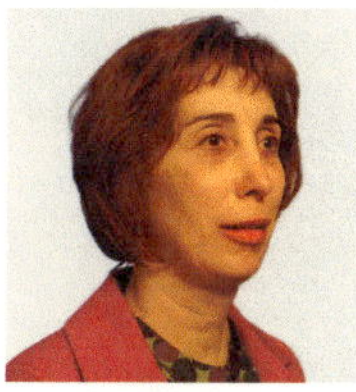

Assoc. Prof. Dr. Daniela Lazar began her career in a center of excellence, the Department of Gastroenterology and Hepatology, University of Medicine and Pharmacy "Victor Babes" Timisoara, Romania, where she acquired clinical skills in gastroenterology, learned the techniques of endoscopy and abdominal ultrasonography and began her research activity. Besides gastroenterology, she showed interest in oncology and the research of gastrointestinal neoplastic conditions, especially gastric cancer. Dr. Lazar is specialized in gastroenterology, medical oncology, and internal medicine. Currently, besides academic and teaching activities, she conducts integrated clinical practice in the Department of Internal Medicine, Emergency Military Clinical Hospital Timisoara. Dr. Lazar obtained a Ph.D. with a thesis on gastric cancer. She has participated in many national and international congresses with research studies in gastroenterology, internal medicine, and digestive oncology. She has published many papers on angiogenesis, premalignant lesions, and prognostic factors in gastric cancer in renowned international journals. She has also published review articles on targeted treatments and immunotherapy in gastric cancer, as well as the impact of artificial intelligence in diagnosing premalignant/malignant esophageal and gastric conditions. She is also interested in the epidemiology, phenotypes, and treatment of inflammatory bowel diseases, being part of the national and international working groups in this domain. Dr. Lazar is the author/co-author of several books and book chapters on different gastroenterological, oncological, and internal medicine topics. Moreover, Dr. Lazar is an academic book editor and a journal reviewer.

Contents

Preface

Helicobacter pylori is a helix-shaped, gram-negative, microaerophilic bacterium that characteristically colonizes the gastric epithelium. It is the most common bacterial infection worldwide, affecting approximately 4.4 billion individuals globally. In recent decades, *H. pylori* has emerged as an important player in the landscape of infectious diseases, profoundly impacting the fields of gastroenterology, microbiology, and clinical medicine. This bacterium, with its unique capacity to colonize the human stomach, has become a major point of research and clinical attention due to its association with a wide array of gastrointestinal diseases, ranging from gastritis and peptic ulcers to more severe conditions like mucosa-associated lymphoid tissue and gastric adenocarcinoma. Moreover, there are many extragastric complications that researchers have associated with *H. pylori* infection, including iron deficiency and vitamin B12 deficiency anemia, diabetes mellitus, and cardiovascular, dermatological, and even certain neurological diseases. Also, an inverse relationship has been advanced, with *H. pylori* having a positive protective role in several diseases including asthma, gastroesophageal reflux disease (GERD), esophageal cancer, Crohn's disease, and other conditions.

For many centuries, the human stomach was considered a hostile environment, resistant to bacterial colonization. Then, in 1983, came the revolutionary discovery of *H. pylori*, a resilient bacterium that defies expectations and develops in the stomach's acidic region. Since then, the story of *H. pylori* has been one of remarkable twists and turns, revealing its profound impact on human health and igniting a quest for deeper understanding. In 2005, the Australian researchers Barry Marshall and Robin Warren were awarded the Nobel Prize in Physiology for their pioneering discovery of the bacterium *H. pylori* and its role in gastritis and peptic ulcer disease. The demonstration of the link between *H. pylori* and peptic ulcer changed the clinical course of this disease; thanks to this knowledge, peptic ulcer transformed from a chronic and disabling disease into a condition that can be cured using a short, combined regimen of antibiotics in association with acid secretion inhibitors.

The World Health Organization (WHO) defined *H. pylori* as a group 1 carcinogen *H. pylori* has been demonstrated as the main risk factor for gastric cancer, with *H. pylori* infection accounting for more than 60% of gastric tumors. Gastric carcinogenesis represents the multistep process in which *H. pylori* infection determines the development of chronic non-atrophic gastritis that can progress to atrophy and intestinal metaplasia, dysplasia, and finally gastric cancer. In the background of this sequential tumorigenic process, both the presence of specific *H. pylori* virulence factors, such as cytotoxin-associated gene A (CagA) and vacuolating cytotoxin A (VacA) along with the persistence of chronic inflammatory response, play a crucial role in producing DNA damage of the host cell and subsequently the activation of specific pathways that induce cell survival and proliferation. Studies show that *H. pylori* eradication effectively reduces the risk of gastric cancer, especially in minority groups that are at higher risk of developing this neoplasia and in areas of high *H. pylori* and gastric cancer prevalence.

This book, *Helicobacter pylori Infection – An Up to Date on the Pathogenic Mechanisms, Diagnosis and Clinical Management*, provides a comprehensive overview of the complexity of this bacterial infection. As editors and contributors, our aim is to provide a thorough exploration of the pathogenesis, diagnostic approaches, and contemporary clinical strategies in managing *H. pylori*-associated diseases.

This book takes the reader on a journey through the multifaceted world of *H. pylori* infection. The first section provides insights into the most recent knowledge of the pathogenesis, virulence factors, and complex adaptive modalities of *H. pylori* that allow this bacterium to colonize the stomach. In this direction, we delve into the intricate pathogenic mechanisms employed by this bacterium to colonize the stomach, evade our immune defenses, and furthermore trigger inflammation. The book explores a diverse spectrum of clinical manifestations, ranging from asymptomatic colonization to peptic ulcers and even stomach cancer.

At the forefront of this narrative lies the evolution of diagnosis and clinical management. From initial breath tests and urea breath tests to cutting-edge molecular techniques, we witness the continuous refinement of tools to identify and eradicate *H. pylori*. The book presents modern indications and treatment regimens for *H. pylori* infection. It also explores the emerging challenges posed by antibiotic resistance and the promise of future therapeutic strategies.

Data regarding *H. pylori* eradication efficiency on the reversibility of premalignant conditions such as atrophy and intestinal metaplasia are contradictory. It is considered that even if this pathogen is successfully treated in patients with chronic atrophic gastritis, regression of atrophy does not always appear. The Maastricht Consensus III report introduced for the first time the phrase "point of no return," after which eradication of *H. pylori* infection no longer offers a significant preventive effect on the development of gastric cancer. This specific step in the gastric carcinogenic process known as the Correa cascade is considered to be the appearance of severe atrophy and intestinal metaplasia. This is why it is essential to search for novel modalities of primary cancer prevention by associating in the complex therapy of this specific category of patients drugs for the restoration and regeneration of the gastric mucosa. The authors present an innovative treatment regimen, suggesting that the inclusion of alpha-glutamyl-tryptophan will offer a superior effect in the sophisticated management of chronic atrophic gastritis associated with *H. pylori* and designated for primary prophylaxis of gastric cancer.

H. pylori infection has been linked with gastric conditions and gastric carcinogenesis for many years, but its extra digestive involvement is still unclear. The second section of our book aims to provide latest information on its potential role in neurological disorders such as Alzheimer's disease, stroke, multiple sclerosis and Parkinson's disease, dermatological diseases such as urticaria, rosacea and psoriasis, ophthalmological disorders such as glaucoma, chorioretinitis and blepharitis, hematologic diseases like anemia, thrombocytopenia and neutropenia as well as cardio-vascular diseases including myocardial infarction, coronary atherosclerosis and hypertension, COVID19, metabolic pathology such as diabetes mellitus and metabolic syndrome, and even autoimmune thyroid diseases.

The current data support the idea that the occurrences of *H. pylori* and Crohn's disease are negatively associated. It has been demonstrated that *H. pylori* induces the change of immune profile, resulting in a specific tolerogenic phenotype, partially responsible for *H. pylori* ability to avoid host immune reactions. Some researchers suggest that *H. pylori* infection may serve as a signal for other gastrointestinal disorders, an aspect that would offer some protection against Crohn's disease. Studies demonstrate that the microbiota in the upper digestive tract differs among individuals who are positive for *H. pylori* vs. those who are negative for *H. pylori*. Research should also be focused on concomitant factors to *H. pylori* infection, such as changes in the gut microbiota, which may have an impact on the etiology of Crohn's disease.

Dermatological diseases including psoriasis are shown by some studies to present a negative correlation with *H. pylori* infection. Psoriasis represents a chronic, immune-mediated inflammatory dermatological condition affecting approximately 125 million individuals globally. Despite the negative correlation described formerly between *H. pylori* and psoriasis, many more recent studies have cancelled the formal facts and proved furthermore that *H. pylori* eradication has a beneficial influence on psoriasis severity.

The background instruments through which *H. pylori* impacts the pathogenesis or influences the severity of a variety of extragastric disorders are extremely complex and only partially understood, but they seem to act by inducing systemic inflammation as the common pathway. *H. pylori* infection leads to the release of several proinflammatory factors such as IL-1, IL-6, TNF, and C-reactive protein, which determine the development of chronic inflammation. Chronic inflammation has been shown to contribute to many chronic disorders affecting different organs and systems, such as cardiovascular, metabolic, dermatologic, and ophthalmic conditions as well as COVID-19 infection. All these mechanisms seem to be similar in most chronic neurological disorders, except for multiple sclerosis (MS). In MS, there is a unique immune response triggered by *H. pylori* infection, resulting in an increase in Treg lymphocytes. Some researchers suggest that this immune shift could benefit patients by slowing down the process of demyelination.

Also, several studies have shown that *H. pylori* eradication treatment may improve symptoms and even have a positive impact on treatment results in certain diseases. Future research is needed and will guide the definition and development of novel and innovative treatment strategies for better management of a multitude of different conditions. Therefore, large-scale prospective studies and molecular research will gather sufficient knowledge in this domain and will offer new perspectives regarding detailed pathogenic mechanisms.

In the context of the presented data, we suggest that doctors and researchers of different specialties should take into consideration the possible presence and implication of *H. pylori* infection. Moreover, they should analyze the potential positive effect of eradication therapy on the course of the specific disease they are studying using fundamental research or that they are managing in their clinical practice. Specialists also have to consider disease risk reduction this treatment might offer.

As editors, we are immensely grateful to our esteemed contributors, whose expertise and dedication have shaped this book into a valuable resource for clinicians, researchers, and students alike. We hope that this comprehensive overview will serve as a guiding light in navigating the complex terrain of *H. pylori* infection, fostering a deeper understanding and ultimately improving patient outcomes.

Daniela Cornelia Lazăr
Associate Professor of Internal Medicine,
Department V of Internal Medicine I,
Discipline of Internal Medicine IV,
"Victor Babeş" University of Medicine and Pharmacy,
Timişoara, Romania

Section 1

Pathogenesis of Helicobacter Infection in the Development of Gastric Conditions Diagnosis and Management

Chapter 1

Helicobacter pylori Gastric Infection: Pathogenesis and Clinical Management

Neha Bisht and Amar P. Garg

Abstract

Helicobacter pylori (H. pylori) is a Gram-negative bacterium that infects approximately 50% of the world population, and currently, no treatment is satisfactory for its management. Understanding the pathophysiology and pathogenesis mechanisms of *H. pylori* has increased over the years. Proper adherence and colonization of *H. pylori* induce genetic alterations, express numerous virulence factors, and trigger diverse adaptive mechanisms, making possible the colonization of an organ with a highly acidic lumen. The mode for the transmission of infection can be oral-oral or fecal-oral. Various effector proteins or toxins are released by the organism for successful colonization and infection. For the virulence and pathogenicity of *H. pylori*, the virulence factors, host, and environmental factors interplay a very important role. Virulence factors for *H. pylori* enhanced the pathogenicity of cytotoxin-associated antigen A, vacuolating cytotoxin, duodenal ulcer promoting gene A protein, outer inflammatory proteins, and gamma-glutamyl transpeptidase. The host immune system through Th1-polarized response plays a crucial role in the course of infection. The most common symptoms in *H. pylori*-positive individuals are peptic ulcers, gastric adenocarcinomas, and mucosa-associated lymphoid tissue lymphomas, whereas some positive individuals remain asymptomatic. Detection of *H. pylori* infection can be through invasive and noninvasive diagnostic methods. We critically reflect on the infection of *H. pylori* and the virulence and pathogenesis mechanisms of *H. pylori*.

Keywords: pathogenesis, virulence factor, colonization, transmission, diagnosis

1. Introduction

Helicobacter pylori (*H. pylori*) is a gram-negative, motile, helical, and microaerophilic (5% O_2, 15% CO_2 & 80% N, required low concentration of O_2 than in the atmosphere) microorganism that is considered as one of the most successful pathogens due to its persistent infection in the human stomach, that inhabits the gastric environment of more than half of the world population of 4.4 billion people worldwide [1–3]. Various shreds of evidence suggest that *H. pylori* are the etiological agent of both extra-gastric and gastric diseases (gastric malignancy, peptic ulcer, chronic gastritis) [4–6]. The main reason for the occurrence of infection among the members of the same family (parents and children) is the route of transmission of *H. pylori* through oral–oral transmission. In this way, during feeding sharing utensils seems to be important for the establishment of infection [7]. Another route for the transmission of infection is fecal-oral, due to the ingestion of contaminated water and unsatisfactory basic sanitation conditions [8]. Improvement of living conditions and socioeconomic status are the two factors that greatly influence the reduction in *H. pylori* infection [9]. It was believed that the gastric environment was sterile because of its high acidity until the discovery of *H. pylori* infection from gastric mucosa by Warren and Marshall's [10, 11]. The bacteria use various mechanisms that provide mobility improvement, robust adherence to epithelial cells, and an enzymatic apparatus that allows the establishment of an appropriate microenvironment for the perpetuation of infection [12–15]. Certain virulence factors are responsible for the potential pathogenicity of infection such as vacuolating cytotoxin (VacA), cytotoxin-associated antigen A (CagA), duodenal ulcer promoting gene A protein (DupA), outer inflammatory protein (OipA) and gamma-glutamyl transpeptidase (GGT) and genetic substrates of the host [*e.g.*, IL1B gene cluster and tumor necrosis factor-α (TNFα) gene polymorphism] play an important role [16–20] shown in **Figure 1**. During the course of infection host immune system play a very pivotal role shown in **Figure 1**. Flagella-mediated motility is used by *H. pylori* for movement toward the epithelial cells of stomachs and penetrating the mucus lining [21]. With all the suitable conditions, organism crosses the acidic environment. At the mucus layer, the coccoid form enabled its colonization [22, 23]. Attachment to the host epithelial cells is through the production of an adhesin [21, 24]. So far colonization of *H. pylori* could be negatively and positively associated with the induction and progression of several diseases [23, 25, 26]. It has been reported to be linked to gastric and duodenal ulcers, gastric carcinoma, and gastric mucosa-associated lymphoid tissue (MALT) lymphoma [6, 27, 28]. Several other studies are also directing a positive correlation between gastrointestinal diseases and *H. pylori*. Many research shows a positive association between *H. pylori*, duodenal ulcer and gastric ulcer [29], gastritis [30], and esophageal cancer [31]. Moreover, evidence shows a positive

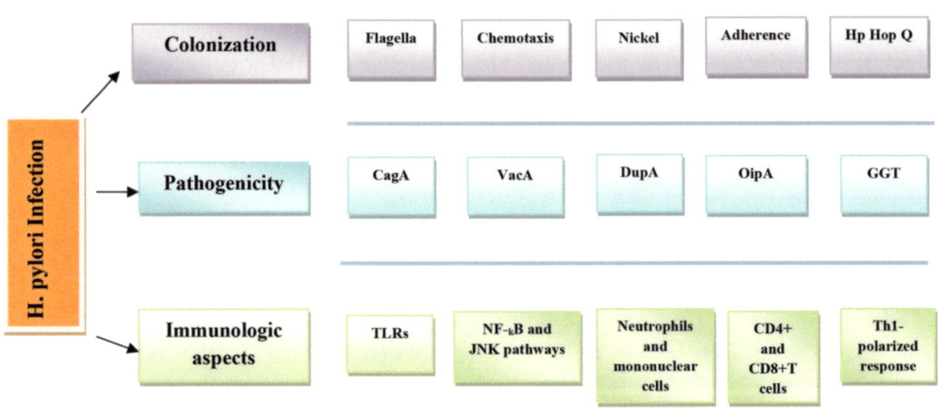

Figure 1.
Representation of characteristics of H. pylori *infection.*

association between *H. pylori* and non-gastrointestinal diseases such as diabetes mellitus [32], coronary artery disease [33], and anemia [34].

2. Clinical manifestations and diagnosis

The discovery of *H. pylori* in the early 1980s caused peptic ulcer diseases [35]. By International Agency for Research on Cancer in 1994 H. pylori was first classified as a carcinogen [36]. In 2001, an epidemiological study stated that patients with H. pylori were nearly six times more potent to develop gastric cancer compared with uninfected people [36]. In 2015, a community of gastroenterologists meticulously recognized *H. pylori* gastritis as an infectious disease and recommended its eradication [37]. This recommendation has repeatedly been confirmed by more recent consensus statements [35, 38, 39]. The most recent consensus conferences on the proactive testing and eradication of *H. pylori* infection [35, 38, 39]. Patients with uninvestigated dyspepsia, having a history of past or current gastric or duodenal ulcer, with a diagnosis of gastric mucosa-associated lymphoid tissue lymphoma, having a family history with peptic ulcer or gastric cancer, and a person with constant use of non-steroidal anti-inflammatory drugs should be recommended for *H. pylori* testing [35, 38]. The strengths and weaknesses of endoscopic and noninvasive tests are shown in **Table 1**.

First-generation immigrants from high-prevalence countries and potential high-risk populations were targeted for testing. Once the presence of the infection has been diagnosed and documented outreach to family members is suggested because transmission from person to person occurs within families [40]. Testing and treating of *H. pylori*-infected individuals can protect other members from infection as well as re-infection from its related diseases [41]. This approach may engage those who test positive to concur with the eradication treatment [41, 42]. To detect *H. pylori* infection a wide variety of methods is available [43]. Because the organism is trophic for gastric epithelium, *H. pylori* are primarily found in the stomach which causes an acute-on-chronic inflammation [44]. Using special stains, organisms can be detected the most accurate and popularly used is immunohistochemistry with *H. pylori*-specific antibodies [45, 46]. Wide range of other tests such as serologic tests for anti–*H. pylori* IgG antibodies and by using molecular testing such as next-generation sequencing [47]. Other tests are noninvasive while some require endoscopy to sample gastric contents, amongst them noninvasive testing is more preferred [48, 49].

The diagnostic strategy utilized clinical indication as well as the local availability and costs of the different tests followed by patient preferences [35]. The presence of the infection gives rise to a serum immune response. Recently, the most commonly used diagnostic test was serology [38]. By Medicare serology is generally neither recommended currently. Tests for the detection of *H. pylori* infection are shown in **Table 1**. IgA and IgM anti–*H. pylori* tests available in some laboratories are not recommended or trusted because of their low specificity and sensitivity generally not approved by the US Food and Drug Administration (FDA). Another important diagnostic method for *H. pylori* is the rapid urease test (RUT). RUT detects an increase in pH of the reagent after the addition of a biopsy specimen that contains *H. pylori* to the reagent [35, 38]. The sort of pH variation is caused by the transformation of the urea test reagent into ammonia. As compared to other tests, RUT is quick, cheap, easy, and specific and is a widely available test [50]. The urea

Tests	Mechanism	Strengths	Weaknesses
Endoscopic			
Culture	Can be kept in a transport medium, like Portagerm pylori or Stuart's transport medium up to 24 h at 4°C. The commonly used media include Pylori agar, Skirrow agar, Columbia blood agar, Brucella agar, Brain heart infusion or Trypticase soy agar, supplemented with sheep or horse blood.	Allows testing of antibiotic susceptibilities	Poor availability in some countries
Molecular-based	Several target genes like UreA, glmM, UreC, 16S rRNA, 23S rRNA, HSP60, and VacA genes detected for the detection of *H. pylori*	Detects infection and can assess susceptibility/resistance for all six commonly used antibiotics. Stool can be used. It gives Rapid results (days)	not to be covered by insurance
Histology	Accuracy of histology, such as the site, size and number of biopsies, the staining methods, proton pump inhibitor (PPI), antibiotics of the examining pathologist.	Can be used for the testing of infection and evaluate for eradication. Provides additional information such as degree of inflammation and associated pathology	Accurate results require interested pathologist and use of special stain, preferably immunohistochemical
Rapid urease	Convert the urea test reagent to ammonia, resulting in increase of pH and color change during pH monitor	It is a Rapid, Inexpensive. Good sensitivity and specificity	Requires prior cessation of antibiotics, bismuth. products, or proton pump inhibitors to reduce risk of false negative results
Noninvasive			
Serology	Detection of Specific anti-*H. pylori* IgG antibodies in the patient's serum	Widely available, Least expensive. Does not require medication modifications prior to testing	Does not reliably delineate between active and previous infection. Cannot confirm eradication
Stool antigen	assesses the presence of bacterial antigens in stool.	High sensitivity and specificity. Can be used to test for active infection and evaluate for eradication	Stool sample needed, patient aversion. Requires prior cessation of antibiotics, bismuth products, or proton pump inhibitors to reduce risk of false negative results
Urea breath	Enzyme splits urea into ammonia and CO_2Patients ingest urea labeled with either 13C or 14C, and the labeled urea comes into contact with the mucosa and diffuses through the mucus towards the *H. pylori* and the mucosal blood supply	High sensitivity and specificity Can be used to test for active infection and evaluate for eradication	Resources and trained personnel needed to reliably reproduce test Requires prior cessation of antibiotics, bismuth products, or proton pump inhibitors to reduce risk of false negative results

Table 1.
Strengths and weakness of endoscopic and noninvasive tests for the detection of H. pylori *infection.*

breadth test (UBT) and the stool antigen test (SAT) are the main non-invasive tests for the diagnosis of active infection [51, 52]. UBT is based on the mechanism of degradation of 13C or 14C-labeled urea into CO_2 that can be measured by an infrared spectrometer [38, 52]. The false positive tests are commonly associated with serology but can occur in the UBT. For example presence of achlorhydria promotes excessive growth of non–*H. pylori* organisms that produce urease result in false positive UBTs. The apparent failure of repeated treatment is the main cause of false positive tests [38, 50, 51]. The apparent failure of repeated treatment results in False positive tests. When false positive tests are suspected, a less expensive option for UBT is with a stool antigen test or endoscopy for the diagnosis of *H. pylori* [51, 53]. For the diagnosis of *H. pylori* infection urine test has been a new promising non-invasive largely recommended as an alternative [51, 54].

A meta-analysis reported that testing for antibodies from urine samples might be a good diagnostic option [54, 55]. For the confirmation of the accuracy of this method, further studies are necessary. Through the discovery of specific serological markers for the diagnosis of *H. pylori*, the infection has been developed. A recent study confirmed the accuracy of the "hook-associated protein 2 homologs", FliD, as a marker of the diagnosis of *H. pylori* infection [54]. The use of Flid ELISA method for the detection of *H. pylori* infection provides up to 99% high specificity and 97% of sensibility at a low cost [35, 41, 51, 56].

3. Pathogenesis

3.1 Colonization

A special mechanism is required by *H. pylori* for successful colonization in the gastric environment. After entering the gastric environment *H. pylori* uses crucial flagellar motility for swimming in gastric content which allows the bacteria to get into the gastric mucus layer [38, 40, 51]. Flagella movements are differ in different media "spreading" in solid media and "swarming" movements, or "swimming motility" in liquid media [57]. Various mutations in genes that encode specific flagellar proteins such as fliD, FlaA, and FlaB disrupts the motility of *H. pylori* resulting in reduce colonization in the gastric mucosal layer [58]. Apart from flagella, the mobility of *H. pylori* lies in the chemotaxis actions of various molecules like mucin, urea, sodium bicarbonate, sodium chloride, and specific amino acids [59]. In recent years various colonization factors like urease, GGT, Flolitin-like protein (FLOT), and RhpA [60]. Several *H. pylori* chemoreceptors like T1pA, B, C, and D, CheA kinase, and various coupling proteins are all important for bacterium colonization [61].

Apart from them, various transition metals are crucial for living organisms, as they serve as cofactors for enzymatic reactions that enhanced the rate of reaction which carries out genetic material replication, transcription, attenuation of oxidative stress, and cellular energy production [54]. In bacteria for survival and successful infection, these metals are crucial [62]. Nickel is an essential metal for *H. pylori* and cofactors for two important enzymes like urease and hydrogenase, both enzymes play a vital role in the process of infection [14]. *H. pylori* urease catalyzes the hydrolysis of urea to ammonia and carbon dioxide which acts as a buffer medium that diminished the acidity of the stomach [63, 64]. Hydrogenase is a signaling cascade that allows Hydrogen as a source of energy for metabolism to be used by *H. pylori* [65]. In the interaction between bacteria and host Adhesion molecules and surface receptors of gastric cells play a very important role [14, 65]. The well-characterized molecule is blood group antigen binding adhesin A (BabA) that carries specific binding to b and H-1 Lewis antigens from the surface of epithelial cells of gastric [66, 67]. The adhesion of the outer membrane Hp HopQ depicts the bacterial-host interaction. These adhesins bind to the cell adhesion molecules related to the carcinoembryonic antigen 1,3,5 and 6 (CEACAMs which give rise to cell signaling mediated by the HopQ-CEACAM interaction that allows the translocation of CagA which is the most crucial and virulence factor of *H. pylori* that increase pro-inflammatory mediators [63, 64, 68–70]. 64 outer membrane proteins (OMPs) of *H. pylori* are grouped into five gene families. *Hop* and *hor* genes are part of family 1, which encodes BabA/B/C, SabA/B, and AlpA/B [64]. In the virulence of *H. pylori,* various OMPs have been identified [64].

3.2 Cytotoxin-associated gene product (CagA)

Cytotoxin-associated gene product (CagA) is one of the most important and studied virulence factors of *H. pylori*. Expression of cagA is always induced whenever the pathogen adhered to the epithelial cells [71]. The cag-pathogenicity island (*cag*PAI) is approximately 40kb that encodes CagA [72], type (IV) secretion system (T4SS) [73], and oncoproteins [74]. CagPA1 is a 40kb chromosomal DNA region of which 31 genes form a type IV secretion system (T4SS) [65, 73]. Seven different secretion systems from I-VII are present, amongst them penetration in the plasma membrane and delivery of bacterial molecules directly to the cytoplasm of the target cells is done by Type III and IV. Flagellum-like tube to translocate effector proteins into eukaryotic host cells performed by type III secretion system (T3SS) whereas a pilus-based structure to mediate the delivery of DNA or proteins into target cells employed by type IV secretion system (T4SS). Cytotoxic effect on the host cell, induced by oncoprotein that is injected into the cell via a pilus formed by the T4SS [74, 75]. This results in the induction of cellular alterations like cellular proliferation, impairing cell motility, apoptosis, and change in the pattern of the cytoskeleton [76].

Transport of CagA protein from gastric mucosal surface to endothelial cells for the tyrosine phosphorylation, carried out by T4SS which directly induces an immune response [75, 77]. The specific interaction between the *H. pylori* HopQ adhesin and the CEACAM (a cellular adhesion molecule) is used for translocating CagA into gastric epithelial cells [77]. Some studies showed this interaction using CEACAM-humanized (hCEACAM) mouse PMNs and humans resulting that *H. pylori* Hop Q-dependent interaction greatly eases the translocation and phosphorylation of CagA. The PMNs positively enhanced the expression of pro-inflammatory chemokines MIP-1-alpha whereas chronic mouse model infection showed downregulation of hCEACAM and -6 receptors on neutrophils [38, 78, 79]. Once CagA, the effector protein of *H. pylori* outreach the host cell it interacts with a diversity of SH2 domains where tyrosine phosphorylation took place (**Table 2**). Site of phosphorylation in *H. pylori* coerce with Glu-Pro-Ile-Tyr-Ala (EPIYA) sequence simultaneously or with closely related sequence located at the N-terminal region and a C-terminal tail [87]. The classification of different subtypes of CagA such as CagA-AB, CagA-ABC, CagA-ABD, or CagA-BD totally based on the composition of the EPIYA-A, EPIYA-B, EPIYA-C, and EPIYA-D motifs [89]. Binding of the host SH2 domain with different EPIYA segments also differs, Among all, the D segment is more harmonious than the C segment and releases the maximum amount of IL-8. [77, 89]. The cytotoxin-associated gene A (*cagA*)-positive

Virulence factors	Functions	References
Arginase	Prevents bacterial killing & T-cell proliferation, Stimulate apoptosis, Impairing of immune responses, Help the *H. pylori* to withstand the acidic environment	[80]
Heat shock proteins	Enhancing adherence to epithelial surfaces, engaged in urease activation, apoptosis and autophagy Control, To maintain the structure and properties of the effector proteins, Protection of cell from reactive oxygen species (ROS),Promotes the production and release of IL-8, TNF-α, and COX-2	[81, 82]
Superoxide dismutase (SOD)	Protection of cell from reactive oxygen species (ROS), colonization enhancement, Inhibiting the production of cytokines, Stimulating the activation of macrophage	[83]
γ-glutamyl-transferase	Facilitating the apoptosis and necrosis, Inducing the release of pro-inflammatory proteins and release of ROS, Stimulate DNA damage	[84]
Lipopolysaccharide	Triggering of signaling pathways, Induction of several inflammatory responses, Induce immune responses, Disrupts the mucus secretion	[85]
Cholesteryl α-glucosyltransferase (αCgT)	Shield *H. pylori* from immunological attack, Stimulates the production of pro-inflammatory proteins (e.g. IL-8),Enhancing the bacterial growth and resistance to antibiotics	[86]
Phospholipase	Activating the signaling pathways (e.g. ERK1/2)and Trigger chronic inflammation, Enhancing the bacterial colonization, Involved in the degradation of lipids and damage to mucus layer	[87, 88]

Table 2.
Important virulence factors in H. pylori.

and *cagA*-negative are the two subclasses of *H. pylori* [88]. The *cagA*-positive is more motile as compared to *cagA* negative [88]. A more severe clinical outcome of *H. pylori* infection, associated with mucosal inflammation is due to the presence of two segments *cag* I and *cag* II [87]. The level of expression of *cagA* differs in *H. pylori* strains. Yeh *et al*, 2019 demonstrate that the *H. pylori* strains which possess Y58/E59 polymorphism in the *cagL* are at higher risk of facilitating gastric cancer [87, 88]. Mutations in genes present in the *cag*PAI totally influence virulence [87].

3.2.1 Non-CagA virulence factors

Impairing gastric homeostasis is the main capacity by other various virulence factors. Vacuolating cytotoxins (VacA) protein and its genes are presents in almost all the strains, promotes pathogenicity of *H. pylori* (**Table 2**). Vacuolation is known to be the creation of vacuoles on a host cell which promotes its pathogenicity by inducing cytotoxicity and apoptosis [90]. It promotes endocytic trafficking disruption, perturbations in mitochondrial, depolarization in plasma membrane potential and various ions like chloride, bicarbonate and urea efflux, and results in the activation of MAP kinases [91, 92]. The activation and suppression of the immune response is prompted by VacA that induce immune tolerance through T cells and antigen-presenting cells. Moreover, this protein also enhances the activation and suppression of the immune response resulting in immune tolerance and persistent infection through its activities on T-cells and antigen-presenting cells [93]. The 140 kDa precursor is produced by VacA which undergoes proteolytic process to produce a toxin of 88 kDa in mass [90]. VacA bind to the epithelial cells with the help of receptor-like protein tyrosine phosphatase alpha and beta (RPTP-α, RPTP-β), sphingomyelin, and density lipoprotein receptor-related protein-1 (LRP-1) [90, 94] also binds to β2 integrin (CD18) receptors [90]. The VacA toxins in amino-terminal is 33KDa and carboxy-terminal 55 kDa that transport into extracellular space by type V secretion pathway, subsequently internalized into endosomal compartments [90, 93, 94]. Several clinical outcomes are due to the different polymorphic forms [94].

The virulence factor promotes gastritis, ulcer, and prolonged infection lead to the cancer development [17, 92]. Duodenal ulcer-promoting gene (DupA) gives a higher acid resistance to the bacterium which promote increase in the production of IL-8 in the gastric mucosa [95]. DupA belongs to the T4SS which integrate conjugative element (ICEHptfs4). VirB4 ATPase homolog is encoded by *dupA* ,linked with gastric ulceration [90, 93] .Pro-inflammatory cytokine secreted by mononuclear cells are induced by *dupA* [96]. The secretions of IL-8 and IL-12 are induced by DupA in the gastric mucosa by gastric epithelial cells in vitro [97]. The biomarkers for peptic ulcers disease is due to *dupA* [98]. Recently a study didn't show any positive correlation between *dupA* and peptic ulcer disease [99]. The increased development of peptic ulcers and gastric cancer totally correlated with the discovery of OipA [96]. OipA is one of the important factor in the outcome of the infection is regulated by "slipped strand mispairing", that depends on the quantity of CT dinucleotide repeats in the5' region of *oip*A [100]. This process determines the functionality and nonfunctionality of OipA that enhance the gastric pathogenicity [100]. OipA change the signaling of β-catenin, proliferation of the cell and decreased the cell-cell junctions [100, 101]. *H. pylori* produce the enzyme GGT which catalyzes the conversion of glutamine into glutamate and finally to ammonia; glutathione into glutamate and cysteinylglycine [102]. It lead to the production of reactive oxygen species (ROS) that induce apoptosis and necrosis [20, 21]. The enzyme inhibits T cell proliferation and dendritic cell differentiation [25, 51, 52]. Patients with peptic ulcers have high GGT activity as compared to the other gastroduodenal disease [90, 96]. Other important virulence factors in *H. pylori* shown in **Table 2**.

3.3 Treatment

No universal regimen for the treatment of *H. pylori* infection. Mostly target the regressing symptomatology and mucosa healing [102]. Since 1997 Maarstricht consensus, proton pump inhibitors (PPI) as standard triple therapy by using a standard dose of 500 mg of clarithromycin and 1g of amoxicillin twice for 7 days as a first-line regimen for the eradication of *H. pylori*. Triple therapy is still recommended as the first line of treatment for *H. pylori* infection in areas with a low rate of clarithromycin according to the European Helicobacter and Microbiota Study Group (EHMSG) [49]. A high dose of clarithromycin resistance lowers the rate for eradication rate of clarithromycin-containing triple therapy like 75% cure rate in Argentina is estimated [103]. A recent study showed that in type 2 diabetic patients the rate of infection eradication is up to 74% [103]. The PPIs, bismuth salt, tetracycline, and metronidazole are complex regimens of Bismuth quadruple therapy, recommended as the second-line or even first-line [104]. According to some previous studies it is stated that the multicenter randomized controlled trials (RCTs) rate of curing of bismuth quadruple therapy is notably high in the standard triple therapy from 90.4%

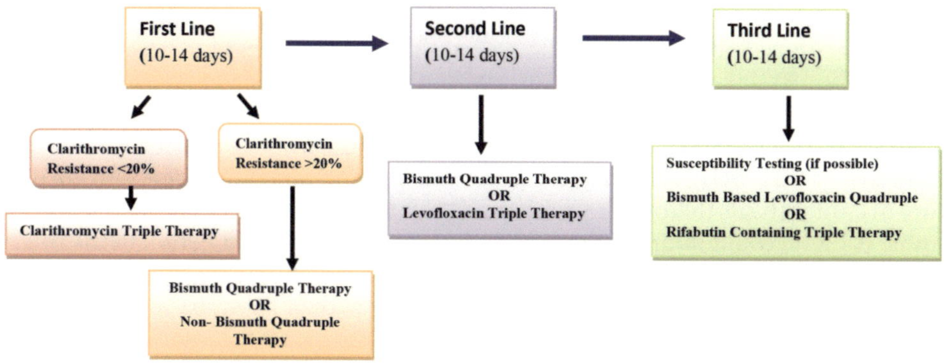

Figure 2.
Treatment regimens of H. pylori *infection.*

to 83.7% for 14 days [103, 104]. In a meta-analysis study, nine RCTs were evaluated and the eradication of infection by bismuth quadruple therapy was the same as those who had received clarithromycin triple therapy [104, 105]. The bismuth quadruple and Levofloxacin triple therapy are the two best therapeutic against infection of *H. pylori* [103]. Levofloxacin regime contains PPIs plus levofloxacin and amoxicillin [104]. Eradication rate of levofloxacin triple therapy (74.5%) and bismuth quadruple therapy (78%) [102, 105]. The third-line therapy is prescribed by using antibiotic susceptibility testing (AST) and prescribed only when the first and second lines of treatment failed [70]. Therapeutic protocols like bismuth-based levofloxacin quadruple therapy or rifabutin triple therapy are used [106]. All three treatment lines are summarized in **Figure 2**.

Probiotics are ——live microorganisms that, when administered in adequate amounts, confer health benefits on the host and they favorably alter the balance in intestinal microflora [107]. Probiotics prevent the adhesion of pathogens by competing for the binding site on intestinal epithelial cells, reducing the colonization of pathogens and thereby preventing the onset of infection. The probiotic's clinical benefits are widely accepted such as diarrhea, antibiotic-associated diarrhea, functional

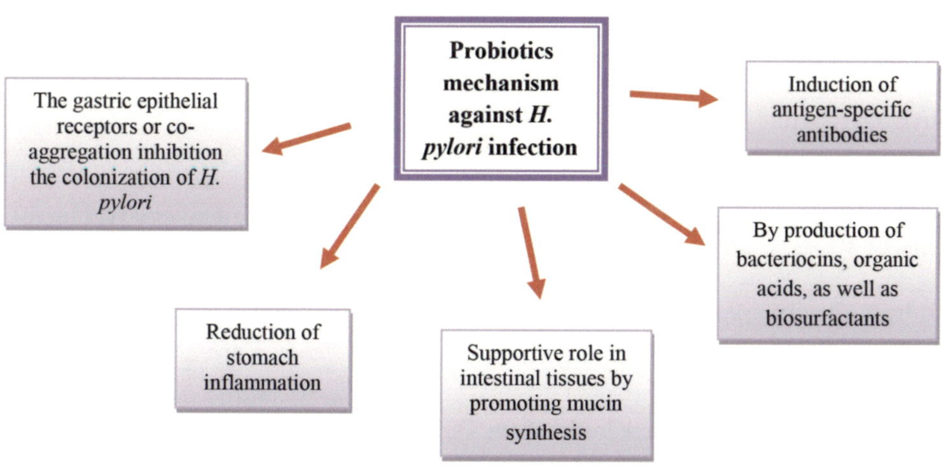

Figure 3.
Mechanism of probiotics against H. pylori infection.

digestive involvements, inflammatory bowel disease, cardiovascular diseases, allergic reactions, and cancer [104, 107]. Anti -*H. pylori* properties proved by spp. of *Lactobacillus* [108]. *Lactobacillus* strains prevent the colonization of *H. pylori* due to their specific adhesins [109] shown in **Figure 3**. The adjuvant therapies with probiotics cure infections caused by *H. pylori* according to the European Helicobacter Pylori Study Group (EHPSG) [104, 105]. *Lactobacillus* spp. and *Bifidobacterium* spp are used more in clinical trials than other probiotics [110]. Studies showed that the yogurt containing bacteria could improve the eradication rate of *H. pylori* infection in the fifth week of treatment [107, 110]. Probiotics act as antibiotic-producing bacteria as they produce antimicrobial substances that inhibit the growth of *H. pylori* [87]. Probiotics' short-chain fatty acids products such as acetic acid, propionic acid, and lactic acid lower the pH of the environment totally unfavorable conditions for the survival of *H. pylori* [111]. Bacteriocins produced by probiotics showed antagonistic activity against *H. pylori* [112]. *Lactobacillus acidophilus* significantly reduced the viability of *H. pylori* [112]. Inhibition of *H. pylori* is due to the antimicrobial Nisin A [113]. The heterogeneous group of antimicrobial proteins is mostly produced by all LAB lactic acid bacteria [114]. Inducing pores in the membrane, activating autolytic enzymes, and downregulating the expression of *vacA*, *cagA*, *luxS*, and *flaA* genes are several mechanisms by bacteriocin to inhibit the growth of *H. pylori* [112, 114].

Author details

Neha Bisht and Amar P. Garg*
Shobhit Institute of Engineering and Technology, Deemed to-be-University, Meerut, India

*Address all correspondence to: amarprakashgarg@yahoo.com

References

[1] Alzahrani S, Lina TT, Gonzalez J, Pinchuk IV, Beswick EJ, Reyes VE. Effect of *Helicobacter pylori* on gastric epithelial cells. World Journal of Gastroenterology. 2014;**20**:12767-12780

[2] Karbalaei M, Khorshidi M, Sisakht-pour B, Ghazvini K, Farsiani H, Youssefi M, et al. What are the effects of IL-1β (rs1143634), IL-17A promoter (rs2275913) and TLR4 (rs4986790) gene polymorphism on the outcomes of infection with *H. pylori* within as Iranian population. Gene Report. 2020;**20**:100735

[3] Hooi JK, Lai WY, Ng WK, Suen MM, Underwood FE, Tanyingoh D, et al. Global prevalence of *Helicobacter pylori* infection: Systematic review and meta-analysis. Gastroenterology. 2017;**153**(2):420-429

[4] Keikha M. Is there a relationship between *Helicobacter pylori* vacA i1 or i2 alleles and development into peptic ulcer and gastric cancer? A meta-analysis study on an Iranian population. New Microbes New Infection. 2020;**36**:100726

[5] Youssefi M, Tafaghodi M, Farsiani H, Ghazvini K, Keikha M. *Helicobacter pylori* infection and autoimmune diseases; Is there an association with systemic lupus erythematosus, rheumatoid arthritis, autoimmune atrophy gastritis and autoimmune pancreatitis? A systematic review and meta-analysis study. Journal of Microbiology, Immunology, and Infection. 2021;**54**(3):359-369

[6] Gravina AG, Zagari RM, De Musis C, Romano L, Loguercio C, Romano M. *Helicobacter pylori* and extragastric diseases: A review. World Journal of Gastroenterology. 2018;**24**(29):3204

[7] Urita Y, Watanabe T, Kawagoe N, Takemoto I, Tanaka H, Kijima S, et al. *Role of infected grandmothers in transmission of Helicobacter pylori to children in a Japanese rural town*. Pediatrician Child Health. 2013;**49**:394

[8] Goh KL, Chan WK, Shiota S, Yamaoka Y. Epidemiology of *Helicobacter pylori* infection and public health implications. Helicobacter. 2011;**16**:1

[9] Laszewicz W, Iwańczak F, Iwańczak B, Task Force of the Polish Society of Gastroenterology; Task Force of the Polish Society of Gastroenterology. Seroprevalence of *Helicobacter pylori* infection in Polish children and adults depending on socioeconomic status and living conditions. Advanced Medical Science. 2014;**59**:147

[10] Warren JR, Marshall B. Unidentified curved bacilli on gastric epithelium in active chronic gastritis. Lancet. 1983;**1**:1273-1275

[11] Wroblewski LE, Peek RM. *Helicobacter pylori*, cancer, and the gastric microbiota. Advanced Experiment in Medical Biology. 2016;**908**:393-408

[12] Eaton KA, Morgan DR, Krakowka S. Motility as a factor in the colonisation of gnotobiotic piglets by *Helicobacter pylori*. Journal of Medical Microbiology. 1992;**37**:123-127

[13] Alm RA, Bina J, Andrews BM, Doig P, Hancock RE, Trust TJ. Comparative genomics of *Helicobacter pylori*: Analysis of the outer membrane protein families. Infectious Immunity. 2000;**68**:4155-4168

[14] Camilo V, Sugiyama T, Touati E. Pathogenesis of *Helicobacter pylori* infection. Helicobacter. 2017;**22**:1

[15] Fischer W. Assembly and molecular mode of action of the *Helicobacter pylori* Cag type IV secretion apparatus. FEBS Journal. 2011;**278**:1203-1212

[16] El-Omar EM, Carrington M, Chow WH, McColl KE, Bream JH, Young HA, et al. Interleukin-1 polymorphisms associated with increased risk of gastric cancer. Nature. 2000;**404**:398-402

[17] Boquet P, Ricci V. Intoxication strategy of *Helicobacter pylori* VacA toxin. Trends in Microbiology. 2012;**20**:165-174

[18] Lu H, Hsu PI, Graham DY, Yamaoka Y. Duodenal ulcer promoting gene of *Helicobacter pylori*. Gastroenterology. 2005;**128**:833-848

[19] Yamaoka Y, Kwon DH, Graham DY. A M(r) 34,000 proinflammatory outer membrane protein (oipA) of *Helicobacter pylori*. Proceedings of the National Academy Science USA. 2000;**97**:7533-7538

[20] Shibayama K, Wachino J, Arakawa Y, Saidijam M, Rutherford NG, Henderson PJ. Metabolism of glutamine and glutathione via gamma-glutamyltranspeptidase and glutamate transport in *Helicobacter pylori*: Possible significance in the pathophysiology of the organism. Molecular Microbiology. 2007;**64**:396-406

[21] Kao C-Y, Sheu B-S, Wu J-J. *Helicobacter pylori* infection: An overview of bacterial virulence factors and pathogenesis. Biomedical Journal. 2016;**39**(1):14-23

[22] Saxena A, Mukhopadhyar AK, Nandi SP. *Helicobacter pylori*: Perturbation and restoration of gut microbiome. Journal of Biosciences. 2020;**45**(1):1-15

[23] Reshetnyak VI, Burnistrov AI, Maev IV. *Helicobacter pylori*: Commensals, symbiont or pathogens? World Journal of Gastroenterology. 2021;**27**(7):545

[24] Huang Y, Wang Q-L, Cheng D-d. Adhesin and invasion of gastric mucosa epithelial cells by *Helicobacter pylori*. Frontiers in Cellular and Infection Microbiology. 2016;**6**:159

[25] Alexander SM, Retnakumar RJ, Chouhan D, Devi TNB, Dharmaseelan S, Devadas K, et al. *Helicobacter pylori* in human stomach: The inconsistencies in clinical outcomes and the probable causes. Frontiers in Microbiology. 2021;**12**:713955

[26] Goni E, Franceschi F. *Helicobacter pylori* and extragastric diseases. Helicobacter. 2016;**1**:45-48

[27] Crowe SE. *Helicobacter pylori* infection. The New England Journal of Medicine. 2019;**380**:1158-1165

[28] McColl KE. *Helicobacter pylori* infection. The New England Journal of Medicine. 2010;**362**(17):1597-1604

[29] Narayanan M, Reddy KM, Marsicano E. Peptic ulcer disease and *Helicobacter pylori* infection. Missouri Medicine. 2018;**115**:219

[30] Watari J, Chen N, Amenta PS, Fukui H, Oshima T, Tomita T, et al. *Helicobacter pylori* associated chronic gastritis, clinical syndromes, precancerous lesions, and pathogenesis of gastric cancer development. World Journal of Gastroenterology: WJG. 2014;**20**:5461

[31] Polyzos SA, Zeglinas C, Artemaki F, Doulberis M, Kazakos E, Katsinelos P, et al. *Helicobacter pylori* infection and esophageal adenocarcinoma: A review

and a personal view. Annals of Gastroenterology. 2018;**31**:8

[32] Chen TP, Hung HF, Chen MK, Lai HH, Hsu WF, Huang KC, et al. *Helicobacter pylori* infection is positively associated with metabolic syndrome in Taiwanese adults: A cross-sectional study. Helicobacter. 2015;**20**:184-191

[33] Yu XJ, Yang X, Feng L, Wang LL, Dong QJ. Association between *Helicobacter pylori* infection and angiographically demonstrated coronary artery disease: A meta-analysis. Experimental and Therapeutic Medicine. 2017;**13**:787-793

[34] Sato Y, Yoneyama O, Azumaya M, Takeuchi M, Sasaki SY, Yokoyama J, et al. The relationship between iron deficiency in patients with *Helicobacter pylori*-infected nodular gastritis and the serum prohepcidin level. Helicobacter. 2015;**20**:11-18

[35] Lee YC, Dore MP, Graham D. Diagnosis and Treatment of *Helicobacter pylori* Infection. Annual Review of Medicine. 2022;**73**:183-195

[36] Aziz F, Chakraborty A, Liu K, Zhang T, Li X, Du R, et al. Gastric tumorigenesis induced by combining *Helicobacter pylori* infection and chronic alcohol through IL-10 inhibition. Carcinogenesis. 2022;**43**:126-139

[37] Sugano K, Tack J, Kuipers EJ, et al. Kyoto global consensus report on *Helicobacter pylori* gastritis. Gut. 2015;**64**:1353-1367

[38] El-Serag HB, Kao JY, Kanwal F, et al. Houston Consensus Conference on testing for *Helicobacter pylori* infection in the United States. Clinical Gastroenterology and Hepatology. 2018;**16**:992-1002

[39] Liou JM, Malfertheiner P, Lee YC, et al. Screening and eradication of *Helicobacter pylori* for gastric cancer prevention: The Taipei global consensus. Gut. 2020;**69**:2093-2112

[40] Bair M-J, Chuang S-L, Lei W-Y, et al. Planning mass eradication of *Helicobacter pylori* infection for indigenous Taiwanese peoples to reduce gastric cancer. Journal of Gastroenterology and Hepatology. 2020;**35**:609-616

[41] Ding S-Z. Global whole family based-*Helicobacter pylori* eradication strategy to prevent its related diseases and gastric cance. World Journal of Gastroenterologia. 2020;**26**:995-1004

[42] Zhao J-B, Yuan L, Yu X-C, et al. Whole family–based *Helicobacter pylori* eradication is a superior strategy to single-infected patient treatment approach: A systematic review and meta-analysis. Helicobacter. 2021;**26**:e12793

[43] Dore MP, Pes GM. What is new in *Helicobacter pylori* diagnosis. An overview. Journal of Clinical Medicine. 2021;**10**:2091

[44] Dixon MF, Genta RM, Yardley JH, Correa P. Classification and grading of gastritis. The updated Sydney System. International Workshop on the Histopathology of Gastritis, Houston 1994. The American Journal of Surgical Pathology. 1996;**20**:1161-1181

[45] Glickman JN, Noffsinger A, Nevin DT, et al. Helicobacter infections with rare bacteria or minimal gastritis: Expecting the unexpected. Digestive and Liver Disease. 2015;**47**:549-555

[46] Lash RH, Genta RM. Routine anti-Helicobacter immunohistochemical staining is significantly superior to reflex staining protocols for the detection of Helicobacter in gastric biopsy specimens. Helicobacter. 2016;**21**:581-585

[47] Pohl D, Keller PM, Bordier V, Wagner K. Review of current diagnostic methods and advances in *Helicobacter pylori* diagnostics in the era of next generation sequencing. World Journal of Gastroenterologia. 2019;**25**:4629-4660

[48] Talley NJ. American Gastroenterological Associationmedical position statement: Evaluation of dyspepsia. Gastroenterology. 2005;**129**:1753-1755

[49] Malfertheiner P, Megraud F, O'Morain CA, et al. Management of *Helicobacter pylori* infection—the Maastricht V/Florence Consensus Report. Gut. 2017;**66**:6-30

[50] Wang YK, Kuo FC, Liu CJ, Wu MC, Shih HY, Wang SS, et al. Diagnosis of *Helicobacter pylori* infection: Current options and developments. World Journal of Gastroenterology. 2015;**21**:11221-11235

[51] Keller J, Hammer HF, Afolabi PR, et al. European guideline on indications, performance and clinical impact of 13C-breath tests in adult and pediatric patients: An EAGEN, ESNM, and ESPGHAN consensus, supported by EPC. United European Gastroenterology Journal. 2021;**9**:598-625

[52] Best LM, Takwoingi Y, Siddique S, et al. Non-invasive diagnostic tests for *Helicobacter pylori* infection. Cochrane Database System Review. 2018;**3**:CD012080

[53] Shimoyama T. Stool antigen tests for the management of *Helicobacter pylori* infection. World Journal of Gastroenterology. 2013;**19**:8188-8191

[54] de Brito BB, da Silva FAF, Soares AS, Pereira VA, Santos MLC, Sampaio MM, et al. Pathogenesis and clinical management of *Helicobacter pylori* gastric infection. World Journal of Gastroenterology. 2019;**25**(37):5578-5589

[55] Gong Y, Li Q, Yuan Y. Accuracy of testing for anti-*Helicobacter pylori* IgG in urine for *H. pylori* infection diagnosis: A systematic review and meta-analysis. BMJ Open. 2017;**7**:e013248

[56] Khalifeh Gholi M, Kalali B, Formichella L, Göttner G, Shamsipour F, Zarnani AH, et al. *Helicobacter pylori* FliD protein is a highly sensitive and specific marker for serologic diagnosis of *H. pylori* infection. International Journal of Medical Microbiology. 2013;**303**:618-623

[57] Gu H. Role of flagella in the pathogenesis of *Helicobacter pylori*. Current Microbiology. 2017;**74**:863-869

[58] Clyne M, Ocroinin T, Suerbaum S, Josenhans C, Drumm B. Adherence of isogenic flagellum-negative mutants of *Helicobacter pylori* and Helicobacter mustelae to human and ferret gastric epithelial cells. Infection Immunity. 2000;**68**:4335-4339

[59] Worku ML, Karim QN, Spencer J, Sidebotham RL. Chemotactic response of *Helicobacter pylori* to human plasma and bile. Journal of Medical Microbiology. 2004;**53**:807-811

[60] Waskito LA, Salama NR, Yamaoka Y. Pathogenesis of *Helicobacter pylori* infection. Helicobacter. 2018;**23**(Suppl. 1):e12516

[61] Aizawa SI, Harwood CS, Kadner RJ. Signaling components in bacterial locomotion and sensory reception. Journal of Bacteriology. 2000;**182**:1459-1471

[62] Becker KW, Skaar EP. Metal limitation and toxicity at the interface between host and pathogen. FEMS Microbiological Review. 2014;**38**:1235-1249

[63] Javaheri A, Kruse T, Moonens K, Mejías-Luque R, Debraekeleer A, Asche CI, et al. *Helicobacter pylori* adhesin HopQ engages in a virulence-enhancing interaction with human CEACAMs. Nature Microbiology. 2016;**2**:16189

[64] Imkamp F, Lauener FN, Pohl D, Lehours P, Vale FF, Jehanne Q, et al. Rapid characterization of virulence determinants in *Helicobacter pylori* isolated from non-atrophic gastritis patients by next-generation sequencing. Journal of Clinical Medicine. 2019;**8**(7):1030

[65] Kalali B, Mejías-Luque R, Javaheri A, Gerhard M. *H. pylori* virulence factors: Influence on immune system and pathology. Mediators Inflammation. 2014;**2014**:426309

[66] Kable ME, Hansen LM, Styer CM, et al. Host determinants of expression of the *Helicobacter pylori* BabA adhesin. Scientific Reports. 2017;**7**:46499

[67] Hansen LM, Gideonsson P, Canfield DR, Boren T, Solnick JV. Dynamic expression of the BabA adhesin and its BabB paralog during *Helicobacter pylori* infection in rhesus macaques. Infection and Immunity. 2017;**85**(6):e00094-e00017

[68] Königer V, Holsten L, Harrison U, Busch B, Loell E, Zhao Q, et al. *Helicobacter pylori* exploits human CEACAMs via HopQ for adherence and translocation of CagA. Nature Microbiology. 2016;**2**:16188

[69] Zhao Q, Busch B, Jiménez-Soto LF, Ishikawa-Ankerhold H, Massberg S, Terradot L, et al. Integrin but not CEACAM receptors are dispensable for *Helicobacter pylori* CagA translocation. PLoS Pathogens. 2018;**14**:e1007359

[70] Chey WD, Leontiadis GI, Howden CW, Moss SF. ACG clinical guideline: Treatment of *Helicobacter pylori* infection. The American Journal of Gastroenterology. 2017;**112**(2):212-239

[71] Chowdhury R. Host cell contact induces fur-dependent expression of virulence factors CagA and VacA in *Helicobacter pylori*. Helicobacter. 2014;**19**(1):17-25

[72] Noto JM Jr, Peek RM. The *Helicobacter pylori*:cag pathogenicity island. Methods in Molecular Biology. 2012;**921**:41-50

[73] Odenbreit S, Puls J, Sedlmaier B, et al. Translocation of *Helicobacter pylori* CagA into gastric epithelial cells by type IV secretion. Science. 2000;**287**:1497-1500

[74] Baj J, Forma A, Sitarz M, Portincasa P, Garruti G, Krasowska D, et al. *Helicobacter pylori* virulence factorsmechanisms of bacterial pathogenicity in the gastric microenvironment. Cell. 2021;**10**(1):27

[75] Altobelli A, Bauer M, Valez K, Cover TL, Muller A. *Helicobacter pylori* VacA targets myeloid cells in the gastric lamina propria to promote peripherally induced regulatory T-cell differentiation and persistent infection. mBio. 2019;**10**:e00261

[76] Machlowska J, Baj J, Sitarz M, Maciejewski R, Sitarz R. Gastric cancer: Epidemiology, risk factors, classification, genomic characteristics and treatment strategies. International Journal of Molecular Sciences. 2020;**21**:4012

[77] Behrens I-K, Busch B, Ishikawa-Ankerhold H, et al. The HopQ-CEACAM interaction controls CagA translocation, phosphorylation, and phagocytosis of *Helicobacter pylori* in neutrophils. MBio. 2020;**11**(1):e03256-ee3319

[78] Bridge DR, Blum FC, Jang S, Kim J, Cha JH, Merrell DS. Creation and initial characterization of isogenic *Helicobacter pylori* CagA EPIYA variants reveals differential activation of host cell signaling pathways. Scientific Reports. 2017;7(1):1-14

[79] Suzuki H, Warren R, Marshal B. *Helicobacter pylori*. Springer. 2016;1:267. DOI: 10.1007/978-4-431-55705-0

[80] Zhang X, Zhang J, Zhang R, Guo Y, Wu C, Mao X, et al. Structural, enzymatic and biochemical studies on *Helicobacter pylori* arginase. The International Journal of Biochemistry & Cell Biology. 2013;**45**(5):995-1002

[81] Dara M, Khashei R, Dehghani B. High frequency of hopQ genotypes among Iranian *Helicobacter pylori* clinical isolates. Le Infezioni in Medicina. 2017;**25**(2):123-126

[82] Feige MH, Sokolova O, Pickenhahn A, Maubach G, Naumann M. HopQ impacts the integrin α5β1-independent NF-κB activation by *Helicobacter pylori* in CEACAM expressing cells. International Journal of Medical Microbiology. 2018;**308**(5):527-533

[83] Švagelj D, Terzić V, Dovhanj J, Švagelj M, Cvrković M, Švagelj I. Superoxide dismutases in chronic gastritis. APMIS. 2016;**124**(4):252-256

[84] Morey P, Meyer TF. The sweeping role of cholesterol depletion in the persistence of *Helicobacter pylori* infections. In: Backert S, editor. Molecular Mechanisms of Inflammation: Induction, Resolution and Escape by *Helicobacter pylori*. Cham: Springer; 2019. pp. 209-227

[85] Zimmermann S, Pfannkuch L, Al-Zeer MA, Bartfeld S, Koch M, Liu J, et al. ALPK1-and TIFA-dependent innate immune response triggered by the *Helicobacter pylori* type IV secretion system. Cell Reports. 2017;**20**(10):2384-2395

[86] Morey P, Pfannkuch L, Pang E, Boccellato F, Sigal M. *Helicobacter pylori* depletes cholesterol in gastric glands to prevent interferon gamma signaling and escape the inflammatory response. Gastroenterology;**154**:1391

[87] Palrasu M, Zaika E, El-Rifai W, et al. Bacterial CagA protein compromises tumor suppressor mechanisms in gastric epithelial cells. The Journal of Clinical Investigation. 2020;**130**(5):2422-2434

[88] Yeh YC, Kuo HY, Chang WL, et al. *H. pylori* isolates with amino acid sequence polymorphisms as presence of both HtrA-L171 & CagL-Y58/E59 increase the risk of gastric cancer. Journal of Biomedical Science. 2019;**26**:4

[89] Hatakeyama M. Anthropological and clinical implications for the structural diversity of the *Helicobacter pylori* CagA oncoprotein. Cancer Science. 2011;**102**(1):36-43

[90] McClain MS, Beckett AC, Cover TL. *Helicobacter pylori* vacuolating toxin and gastric cancer. Toxins. 2017;**9**(10):316

[91] Foegeding NJ, Caston RR, McClain MS, Ohi MD, Cover TL. An overview of *Helicobacter pylori* VacA toxin biology. Toxins. 2016;**8**(6):173

[92] Ricci V. Relationship between VacA toxin and host cell autophagy in *Helicobacter pylori* infection of the human stomach: A few answers, many questions. Toxins. 2016;**8**(7):203

[93] Djekic A, Müller A. The Immunomodulator VacA Promotes Immune Tolerance and Persistent

Helicobacter pylori Infection through Its Activities on T-Cells and Antigen-Presenting Cells. Toxins (Basel). 2016;**8**:2

[94] Yahiro K, Hirayama T, Moss J, Noda M. New insights into VacA intoxication mediated through its cell surface receptors. Toxins. 2016;**8**(5):152

[95] Muzahhed M. *Helicobacter pylori* oncogenicity: Mechanism, prevention and risk factors. Science World Journal. 2020

[96] Jiang X, Xu Z, Zhang T, Li Y, Li W, Tan H. Wholegenome- based *Helicobacter pylori* Geographic surveillance: Visualized and expanded webtool. Frontiers in Microbiology. 2019;**12**:687259

[97] Dadashzadeh K. Relevance of *Helicobacter pylori dupA* and *oipA* genotypes and development of gastric disease. Biomedical Research. 2017;**28**(19):8179-8183

[98] Pereira WN, Ferraz MA, Zabaglia LM, de Labio RW, Orcini WA, Bianchi Ximenez JP, et al. Association among *H. pylori* virulence markers dupA, cagA and vacA in Brazilian patients. Journal of Venomous Animals and Toxins Including Tropical Diseases. 2014;**20**(1):1

[99] Idowu A, Mzukwa A, Harrison U, Palamides P, Haas R, Mbao M, et al. Detection of *Helicobacter pylori* and its virulence genes (cagA, dupA, and vacA) among patients with gastroduodenal diseases in Chris Hani Baragwanath Academic Hospital. South Africa BMC gastroenterology. 2019;**19**(1):1-10

[100] Sallas ML, Dos Santos MP, Orcini WA, David ÉB, Peruquetti RL, Payão SLM, et al. Status (on/off) of oipA gene: Their associations with gastritis and gastric cancer and geographic origins. Archives in Microbiology. 2019;**201**:93-97

[101] Farzi N, Yadegar A, Aghdaei HA, Yamaoka Y, Zali MR. Genetic diversity and functional analysis of oipA gene in association with other virulence factors among *Helicobacter pylori* isolates from Iranian patients with different gastric diseases. Infectious Genetic Evolution. 2018;**60**:26-34

[102] Safavi M, Sabourian R, Foroumadi A. Treatment of *Helicobacter pylori* infection: Current and future insights. World Journal of Clinical Cases. 2016;**4**:5-19

[103] Yao C-C, Kuo C-M, Hsu C-N, Yang S-C, Wu C-K, Tai W-C, et al. First-line *Helicobacter pylori* eradication rates are significantly lower in patients with than those without type 2 diabetes mellitus. Infectious Drug Resistant. 2019;**12**:1425

[104] Zagari RM, Rabitti S, Eusebi LH, Bazzoli F. Treatment of *Helicobacter pylori* infection: A clinical practice update. European Journal of Clinical Investigation. 2018;**48**(1):e12857

[105] Chen PY, Wu MS, Chen CY, Bair MJ, Chou CK, Lin JT, et al. Systematic review with meta-analysis: The efficacy of levofloxacin triple therapy as the first-or second-line treatments of *Helicobacter pylori* infection. Alimentary Pharmacology & Therapeutics. 2016;**44**(5):427-437

[106] Flores-Trevino S, Mendoza-Olazaran S, Bocanegra-Ibarias P. *Helicobacter pylori* drug resistance: Therapy changes and challenges. Expert Review of Gastroenterology & Hepatology. 2018;**12**(8):819-827

[107] Bisht N, Garg AP. Isolation, characterization and probiotic value of lactic acid bacteria from milk and milk products. An International Journal of Biological Sciences. 2019;**9**:54

[108] Yousefi B, Eslami M, Ghasemian A, Kokhaei P, Sadeghnejhad A. Probiotics can really cure an autoimmune disease? Gene Report. 2019;**15**:100364

[109] Iqbal U, Khara HS, Akhtar D, Hu Y, Anwar H, Haq KF, et al. Safety and efficacy of Nitazoxanide-based regimen for the eradication of *Helicobacter pylori* infection: A systematic review and meta-analysis. Gastroenterology Research. 2020;**13**(6):260

[110] Keikha M, Karbalaei M. Probiotics as the live microscopic fighters against *Helicobacter pylori* gastric infections. BMC Gastroenterology. 2021;**21**:388

[111] Boyanova L, Gergova G, Markovska R, Yordanov D, Mitov I. Bacteriocinlike inhibitory activities of seven Lactobacillus delbrueckii subsp. Bulgaricus strains against antibiotic susceptible and resistant *Helicobacter pylori* strains. Letters in Applied Microbiology. 2017;**65**(6):469-474

[112] Negash AW, Tsehai BA. Current applications of Bacteriocin. Int J Microbiol. 2020;**2020**:1-7

[113] Lim E-S. Purification and characterization of two bacteriocins from Lactobacillus brevis BK11 and Enterococcus faecalis BK61 showing anti-*Helicobacter pylori* activity. Journal of Korean Society for Applied Biological Chemistry 2015;58(5):703-714.

[114] Rezaee P, Kermanshahi RK, Falsafi T. Antibacterial activity of lactobacilli probiotics on clinical strains of *Helicobacter pylori*. Iranian Journal of Basic Medical Sciences. 2019;**22**(10):1118

Chapter 2

Alpha-Glutamyl-Tryptophan in the Treatment of Chronic Atrophic Gastritis, Associated with *Helicobacter pylori*

Yury P. Uspensky, Natalia V. Baryshnikova, Yulia A. Fominykh, Alexey A. Krasnov, Sergey V. Petlenko and Vera A. Apryatina

Abstract

To evaluate the effectiveness of alpha-glutamyl-tryptophan as a cytoprotector in comparison with the control group (placebo) as part of the complex therapy of chronic atrophic *H. pylori* (HP)-associated gastritis. A total of 121 patients with chronic atrophic HP-associated gastritis were observed in 3 research centers. Before and after treatment blood test “Gastropanel”, stomach endoscopy with biopsies of atrophied mucosa for histological examination, rapid urease test for *H. pylori* detection, and daily pH-metry were performed. After HP eradication, according to randomization, the study drug (n = 61) or placebo (n = 60) was administered twice a day, in the morning 20–30 minutes before meals and in the evening before bedtime for 28 days. Alpha-glutamyl-tryptophan intake is associated with a statistically significant increase in acidity index according to pH-metry ($p = 0.001$), an increase in the ratio of pepsinogen I/pepsinogen II ($p = 0.003$), decrease in the level of gastrin-17 ($p = 0.005$), increase in the number of glands per 1 mm^2 of the gastric mucosa ($p = 0.028$). Alpha-glutamyl-tryptophan in the treatment of chronic atrophic HP-associated gastritis has a superior regenerative effect compared with placebo, and promotes the restoration of acid-forming and pepsin-forming functions of the stomach.

Keywords: chronic atrophic gastritis, *Helicobacter pylori*, alpha-glutamyl-tryptophan, atrophy, stomach

1. Introduction

In accordance with the current standards for the treatment of chronic gastritis, eradication of *Helicobacter pylori* is an effective strategy to reduce the risk of developing stomach cancer [1–4]. However, a large percentage of *H. pylori*-infected patients get to the primary doctor’s appointment already at the stage of not superficial active gastritis, but at the stage of atrophic gastritis, when the risk of cancer becomes higher [5–8]. Data on the possibility of reverse development of atrophy and intestinal metaplasia after eradication of infection are contradictory [1, 9]. Even if the pathogen is successfully eradicated in patients with chronic atrophic gastritis, regression of atrophy does not always take place. Already the Maastricht Consensus III introduced the term "point of no return", after which *H. pylori* eradication no longer gives a significant preventive effect on the development of stomach cancer [10]. This "point of no return" is considered to be the presence of severe atrophy and intestinal metaplasia. Thus, in a meta-analysis of 12 studies involving 2658 patients conducted by J. Wang et al., it was shown that *H. pylori* eradication reduces atrophy in the stomach body ($p = 0.006$), but not in its antrum ($p = 0.06$), and does not affect intestinal metaplasia in these departments (respectively, $p = 0.42$ and $p = 0.76$) [11]. Consequently, the changes described in the Correa cascade can progress even in the absence of a microorganism, which once again emphasizes the need for additional measures to preserve the structure and function of the gastric mucosa at the stage of atrophy development. Therefore, it is extremely important to look for ways of primary cancer prevention by including in the complex therapy of this category of patients drugs for the restoration of the gastric mucosa, i.e., having a regenerative effect [12]. One of such medicine is alpha-glutamyl-tryptophan. The pharmacological properties of alpha-glutamyl-tryptophan revealed during experimental [13] and clinical [14] studies indicate the effect of this peptide on the unified pathogenetic mechanisms of inflammatory diseases of the gastrointestinal tract: it is effective against chronic gastritis accompanied by atrophic processes of the gastric mucosa [15].

The aim is to evaluate the effectiveness of alpha-glutamyl-tryptophan as a cytoprotector in comparison with the control group (placebo) as part of the complex therapy of chronic atrophic *H. pylori*-associated gastritis.

2. Materials and methods

2.1 Patients population

We included in the study 152 adult patients with a history of diagnosis of "chronic atrophic gastritis" in three research centers. A total of 121 patients met all inclusion criteria: signed informed consent (before the start of the study procedures); men and women aged 40–70 years; previously diagnosed chronic atrophic gastritis; the presence of complaints and symptoms characteristic of chronic atrophic gastritis; confirmed diagnosis of atrophic gastritis associated with *H. pylori* infection by endoscopic and histological examination; hypo- or anacidity according to pH-metry (pH greater than 5.0); negative pregnancy test; use of any methods of contraception during the entire time of participation in the study. Four weeks before participation in the study some drugs are prohibited to use: cytostatic, immunosuppressive, hormonal (hormone-like), antimicrobial or sedative effects, as well as drugs or biologically active additives for the treatment of inflammatory diseases of the stomach, duodenum (bismuth-containing drugs, proton pump inhibitors, antacids, gastric secretion or motility stimulants, antiemetics, laxatives, etc.), liver and pancreas (hepato-pancreatoprotectors, enzymes, choleretics, cholekinetics, etc.), nonsteroidal anti-inflammatory drugs (NSAIDs).

2.2 Diagnostic methods

Before and after treatment complex diagnostic examination was performed for all patients.

Evaluation of the results of daily pH-metry. In the course of the study, the data of the daily pH-metry of the stomach was analyzed twice (before the appointment of the studied drug during the screening period and after taking the course of the studied drug). The analysis included an assessment of the parameters: the minimum pH value, the average pH value, the aggressiveness index, and the acidity index.

Evaluation of the results of histological examination. Morphological (morphometric) analysis of the biopsy data of the gastric mucosa taken from the center of the atrophy zone twice (before the appointment of the test drug during the screening period and after taking the course of the study drug/placebo). The analysis included an assessment of such parameters as the number of glands per 1 mm^2 of the gastric mucosa, the depth of the glands of the gastric mucosa, and the number of lining cells per 100 epithelial cells of the gastric mucosa.

Evaluation of the dynamics of laboratory parameters. "Gastropanel" is a comprehensive study with the determination of a number of biochemical markers associated with gastric secretion and regenerative processes in the gastric mucosa, as well as antibodies to *H. pylori*. The "Gastropanel" complex was performed according to the standard protocol of the manufacturer (BioHit, Finland) and included an assessment of the level of pepsinogen I (PG I), pepsinogen II (PG II), gastrin-17, and the IgG titer to *H. pylori*. In addition to analyzing data on the content of the listed compounds, the PG I/PG II ratio was calculated and analyzed to assess the degree of atrophy. The study was conducted twice (before the appointment of the study drug during the screening period and after the end of the course of taking the study drug/placebo). The ratio of PG1/PG2 decreases linearly with increasing severity of atrophic gastritis.

Verification of the presence of H. pylori infection was made using several methods:

1. A biochemical rapid urease test.

2. Histological examination (Romanovsky-Giemsa staining).

3. A blood test for the presence of antibodies to IgG *H. pylori* was performed in a complex of laboratory tests "Gastropanel".

2.3 Treatment

The order of randomization: patients who met the inclusion criteria and did not have non-inclusion criteria were randomized into two groups: the main and control in a ratio of 1:1. Then performing the randomization procedure, the random number method was used. A double-blind method was used: neither the patients nor the research doctor knew which drug alpha-glutamyl-tryptophan or placebo the study participant received. These measures made it possible to minimize the influence of the human factor and contributed to obtaining more reliable data on the safety and effectiveness of the drug. The study drug and placebo were identical in packaging, labeling, and appearance.

The therapy in the study consisted of two stages:

1. A standard course of eradication therapy with Omeprazole 20 mg two times a day 10 days; amoxicillin 1000 mg two times a day for the first 5 days; clarithromycin 500 mg two times a day for next 5 days.

2. After *H. pylori* eradication, according to randomization, the study drug (n = 61) or placebo (n = 60) was administered twice a day, in the morning 20–30 minutes before meals and in the evening before bedtime for 28 days.

In the patients included in the study, the use of other medications and non-drug treatments other than the use of eradication therapy and the study drug/placebo was not allowed for the treatment of the underlying disease (atrophic gastritis).

During the study, all possible adverse events were recorded.

3. Statistical data processing

The statistical software package "Statistica 12.0 for Windows" was used for statistical analysis. The value $p<0.05$ is taken as the level of statistical significance. The data, the distribution of which corresponded to normal, were presented in the form of arithmetic averages indicating standard square deviations ($M \pm \sigma$). The data, the distribution of which differed from the normal, were presented in the form of median and quartile intervals (Mediana: [25 quartile; 75% quartile]). The Lillefors criterion was used to determine the degree of difference between the distribution and the normal one.

Due to the small sample size, nonparametric criteria were used in most cases to assess the dynamics of indicators between visits. The dynamics of the indicators were evaluated using the Wilcoxon criterion, as well as the McNemar criterion. If necessary, Bonferroni's correction for the multiplicity of comparison was used. The reliability of the differences between the indicators of dependent groups for parametric data with a normal distribution was evaluated using the Student's t-test for dependent samples.

The results of each assessment were considered as statistical indicators of the effect. In the future, the difference in the proportion of patients with a positive effect was calculated according to the primary (main variable) and secondary efficiency parameters, and a two-sided 95% confidence interval was built for this difference. To assess the effectiveness of the studied drug, a statistical analysis of the population according to the protocol (PP) was used.

The study was conducted in strict accordance with the ethical principles of the Helsinki Declaration of the World Medical Association of 1964, as amended in 2013, in accordance with the international standards of the Guidelines for Good Clinical Practice (ICH GCP R2) and other necessary regulatory documents in force on the territory of the Russian Federation.

4. Results

4.1 Data of histological examination

One of the main morphological signs of atrophic gastritis is a decrease in the number of glands of the gastric mucosa, as well as a violation of their histological structure. Therefore, an important indicator for assessing the regenerative effect of alpha-glutamyl-tryptophan can be considered an increase of 26.1% in the number of glands per 1 mm^2 while taking the study drug (**Figure 1**).

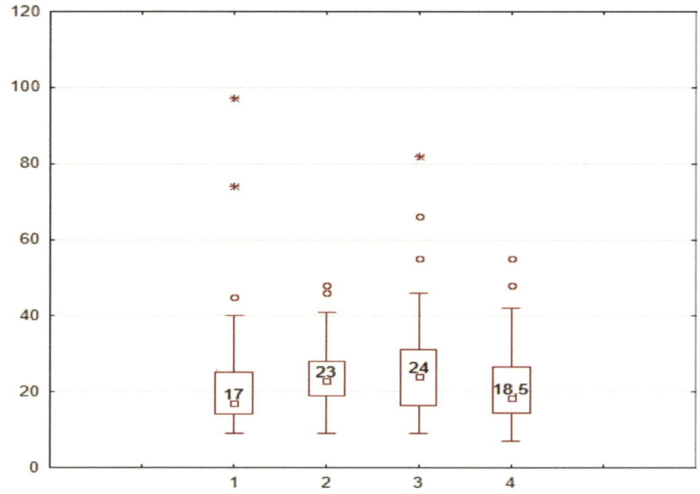

Figure 1.
Diagram of the scale of the dynamics of the number of glands per 1 mm² of the gastric mucosa during the administration of the alpha-glutamyl-tryptophan and placebo.

The medians, 25 and 75% quartiles, outliers of values, and minimum and maximum values of the indicator are presented

Along the abscissa axis of the treatment group:

1. results of alpha-glutamyl-tryptophan group before treatment

2. results of alpha-glutamyl-tryptophan group after treatment

3. results of placebo group before treatment

4. results of placebo group after treatment

On the ordinate axis: the number of glands per 1 mm^2 of the gastric mucosa in the atrophy zone

The diagram shows that taking of alpha-glutamyl-tryptophan leads to the statistically significant ($p = 0.028$) increase in the number of glands per 1 mm^2 of the gastric mucosa in comparison with the initial screening indicators. In the group of patients taking placebo, on the contrary, there was a decrease in the number of glands per 1 mm^2 of the gastric mucosa after the end of treatment in comparison with screening indicators, which had no statistical significance of differences. Intergroup comparison of the final treatment parameters showed that after a course of therapy in patients taking the alpha-glutamyl-tryptophan, the number of glands per 1 mm^2 of the gastric mucosa was statistically significantly higher compared with the results in the placebo group ($p = 0.013$).

4.2 Data of daily pH-metry

The average pH value after taking of study drug was shift in the acidic side by 1.59 times compared to the initial values from 4.3 [2.6; 6.1] to 2.7 [1.6; 4.7] ($p = 0.001$). No statistically significant dynamics of the mean pH was obtained in placebo group: from 4.35 [2.4; 6.1] to 3.6 [1.8; 5.0].

The value of the acidity index increased statistically significantly after taking the study drug as compared with the initial values by 5.44 times (from 8.95 [0; 50.33] to 48.70 [0; 110.90]), ($p = 0.001$), and in comparison with the placebo group by 2.94 times (from 22.80 [0; 63.62] to 16.55 [0; 77.68]), ($p = 0.034$) (**Figure 2**). In the placebo group, a decrease in the acidity index was noted, which indicates the absence of regression of atrophy even against the background of successful eradication of *H. pylori*.

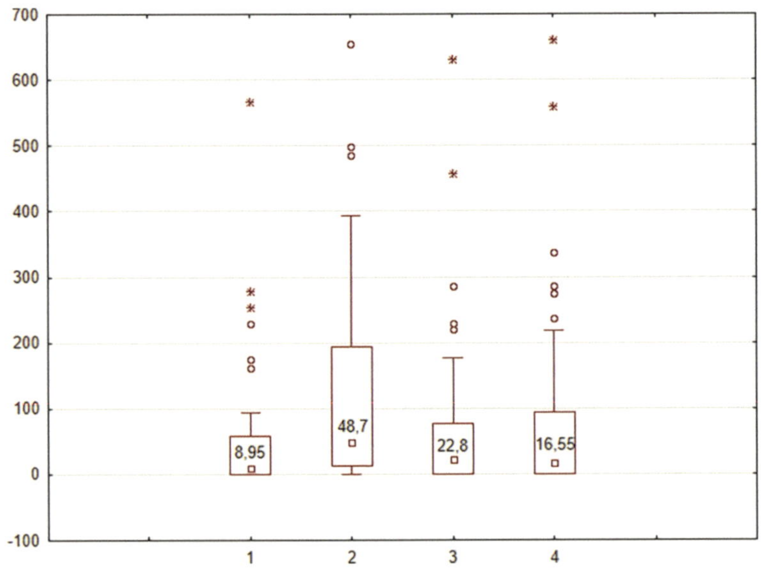

Figure 2.
Diagram of the magnitude of changes in the acidity index of gastric juice during the administration of alpha-glutamyl-tryptophan and placebo.

The medians, 25 and 75% quartiles, outliers of values, and minimum and maximum values of the indicator are presented

Along the abscissa axis of the treatment group:

1. results of alpha-glutamyl-tryptophan group before treatment

2. results of alpha-glutamyl-tryptophan group after treatment

3. results of placebo group before treatment

4. results of placebo group after treatment

On the ordinate axis: stomach acidity index, units

A statistically significant increase in the aggressiveness index by 1.48 times was revealed after taking the study drug when comparing the results before and after treatment (from 4.8 [3.1; 6.2] to 3.25 [1.7; 5.0]), ($p < 0.001$). For the placebo group, the same indicator was 1.18 times (parameter change from 4.9 [2.7; 6.2] to 4.15 [2.0; 5.5]). The effect of the studied drug on the value of the aggressiveness index was more pronounced and stable than that of placebo.

There were no statistically significant changes in the minimum pH of gastric juice during the administration of both the study drug and placebo.

The results obtained indicate that alpha-glutamyl-tryptophan has a clinically significant moderate positive effect on increasing the acidity of gastric juice, i.e. restoring the functional activity of the glandular apparatus of the gastric mucosa in patients with chronic atrophic gastritis, associated with *H. pylori*. These changes in acid secretion can be regarded as an effect that occurs indirectly due to the restoration of the morphological structure of the gastric mucosa. It should be understood that a relatively short course of the drug was used in the study, which, nevertheless, revealed a statistically significant positive effect on the indicators of acid secretion in this category of patients.

4.3 "Gastropanel" data

When evaluating the results of the Gastropanel complex of laboratory examinations, we saw a statistically significant ($p = 0.003$) 1.45-fold increase in the ratio of pepsinogen I /pepsinogen II (PG I/PG II): 9.33 [5.5; 12.2] was revealed in comparison with the initial data (6.43 [4.17; 9.6]) in alpha-glutamyl-tryptophan group and the absence of similar differences in the placebo group (before taking placebo: 7.01 [4.55; 10.9], after taking placebo: 8.03 [4.8; 11.6]) (**Figure 3**).

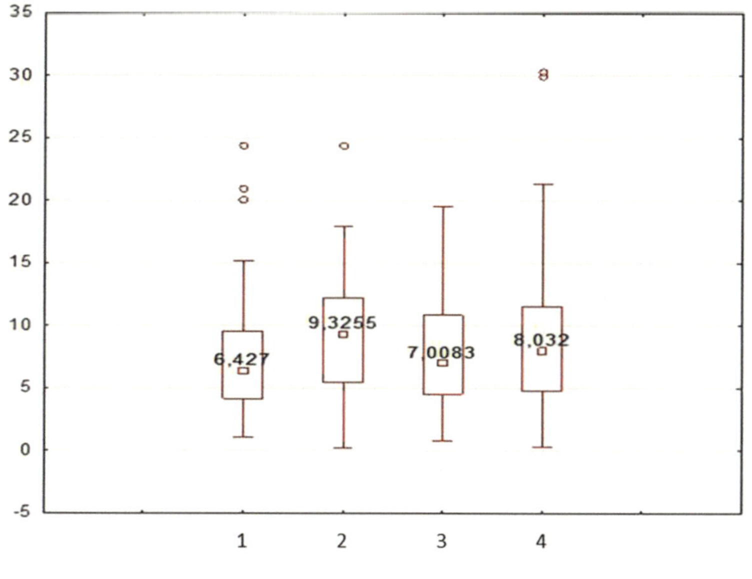

Figure 3.
Diagram of the range of values of the PGI/PGII coefficient in the process of taking alpha-glutamyl-tryptophan and placebo.

The medians, 25 and 75% quartiles, outliers of values, and minimum and maximum values of the indicator are presented

Along the abscissa axis of the treatment group:

1. results of alpha-glutamyl-tryptophan group before treatment

2. results of alpha-glutamyl-tryptophan group after treatment

3. results of placebo group before treatment

4. results of placebo group after treatment

On the ordinate axis: values of the PGI / PGII coefficient, units

The restoration of the normal PGI / PGII ratio indirectly indicates the restoration of pepsin-forming function of the stomach and is an important point in the pathogenetic treatment of chronic atrophic gastritis, since such an effect can be classified as anti-oncogenic.

We found a statistically significant (p = 0.005) 1.75-fold decrease in the level of gastrin-17 in the blood (pmol/L) (2.9 [1.4; 8.6]) in comparison with the initial data (5.1 [1.85; 14.0]) after taking the alpha-glutamyl-tryptophan and the absence of similar differences in the placebo group (before taking placebo: 5.13 [1.38; 16.9]; after taking placebo: 3.14 [1.28; 15.1]) (**Figure** 4). This indicates a decrease in inflammation associated with *H. pylori* invasion. That is, it can be a manifestation of both regenerative and anti-inflammatory effects of alpha-glutamyl-tryptophan.

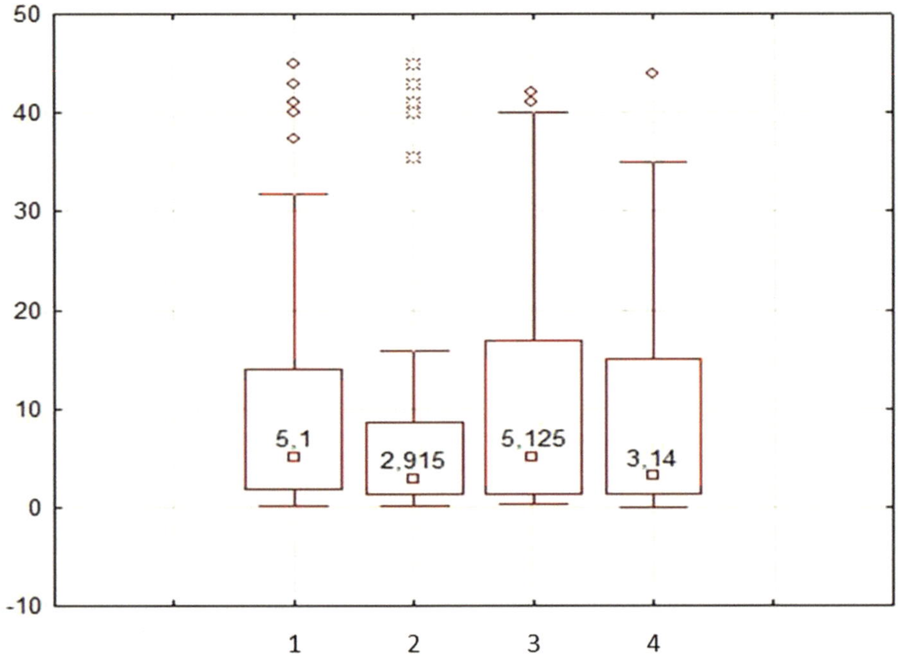

Figure 4.
Diagram of the range of gastrin-17 levels in venous blood (pmol/l) in the process of taking alpha-glutamyl-tryptophan and placebo.

The medians, 25 and 75% quartiles, outliers of values, and minimum and maximum values of the indicator are presented

Along the abscissa axis of the treatment group:

1. results of alpha-glutamyl-tryptophan group before treatment

2. results of alpha-glutamyl-tryptophan group after treatment

3. results of placebo group before treatment

4. results of placebo group after treatment

On the ordinate axis: gastrin-17 level in venous blood, pmol/l

4.4 Estimation of adverse events

In the study, 45 adverse events (AE) were registered. Of these, 20 were on the background of taking the study drug, 12 were on the background of taking a placebo, 13 occurred before the taking of the study drug/placebo. An intergroup comparison of the number of AE detected during the period of taking the study drug and placebo revealed no statistically significant differences ($\chi 2 = 1.55$; $p = 0.213$) in the amount of AE in the study groups. No any serious AE was detected in the study.

5. Conclusion

According to the results of the study, it can be concluded that the study drug alpha-glutamyl-tryptophan, in comparison with placebo, has superior regenerative efficiency (an increase in the number of glands per 1 mm^2 of the gastric mucosa, an increase in the acidity index and a shift in the average pH value to the acidic side according to the daily pH-metry, an increase in the ratio of PG I / PG II and a decrease in the level of gastrin-17 in the blood according to the Gastropanel complex). The study drug promotes the restoration of acid-forming and pepsin-forming functions of the stomach in the treatment of chronic atrophic gastritis in patients aged 40–70 years. It can be assumed that the study drug, due to the restoration of anatomical and functional parameters of the gastric mucosa, also decreases the pro-oncogenic processes associated with the development of atrophy.

Therefore, it can be recommended to include alpha-glutamyl-tryptophan in the complex therapy of chronic atrophic gastritis, associated with *H. pylori* and for primary prophylaxis of gastric cancer. In the future, it is important to conduct studies with the estimation of alpha-glutamyl-tryptophan efficacy in the treatment of chronic atrophic gastritis not associated with *H. pylori*, peptic ulcer disease (*H. pylori*-associated and not associated), chronic non-atrophic gastritis (*H. pylori*-associated and not associated) for improving regeneration of gastric mucosa.

Author details

Yury P. Uspensky[1,2], Natalia V. Baryshnikova[1,2,3*], Yulia A. Fominykh[1,2], Alexey A. Krasnov[4], Sergey V. Petlenko[5] and Vera A. Apryatina[6]

1 St. Petersburg State Pediatric Medical University, St. Petersburg, Russia

2 Pavlov First St. Petersburg State Medical University, St. Petersburg, Russia

3 Institute of experimental Medicine, St. Petersburg, Russia

4 The Herzen State Pedagogical University of Russia, St. Petersburg, Russia

5 Golikov Research Clinical Center of Toxicology under the Federal Medical-Biological Agency, St. Petersburg, Russia

6 Saint Petersburg State University, Institute of translational biomedicine, Universitetskaya Embankment, St. Petersburg, Russia

*Address all correspondence to: baryshnikova_nv@mail.ru

References

[1] Malfertheiner P, Megraud F, O'Morain CA, Gisbert JP, Kuipers EJ, et al. Management of *Helicobacter pylori* infection—the Maastricht V/Florence Consensus Report. Gut. 2017;**66**:6-30

[2] Sugano K, Tack J, Kuipers EJ, Graham DY, El-Omar EM, Miura S, et al. Faculty members of Kyoto Global Consensus Conference. Kyoto global consensus report on *Helicobacter pylori* gastritis. Gut. 2015;**64**(9):1353-1367

[3] Waldum H, Fossmark R. Gastritis, gastric polyps and gastric cancer. International Journal of Molecular Science. 2021;**22**(12):6548

[4] Ansari S, Yamaoka Y. *Helicobacter pylori* virulence factors exploiting gastric colonization and its pathogenicity. Toxins (Basel). 2019;**11**(11):677

[5] Correa P. *Helicobacter pylori* and gastric carcinogenesis. American Journal of Surgery Pathology. 1995;**19**(Suppl. 1): S37-S43

[6] Correa P. Gastric cancer: Overview. Gastroenterological Clinical North America. 2013;**42**(2):211-217

[7] Kishikawa H, Ojiro K, Nakamura K, Katayama T, Arahata K, Takarabe S, et al. Previous Helicobacter pylori infection-induced atrophic gastritis: A distinct disease entity in an understudied population without a history of eradication. Helicobacter. 2020;**25**(1):e12669

[8] Shichijo S, Hirata Y. Characteristics and predictors of gastric cancer after *Helicobacter pylori* eradication. World Journal of Gastroenterology. 2018;**24**(20):2163-2172

[9] Watari J, Chen N, Amenta PS, Fukui H, Oshima T, Tomita T, et al. Helicobacter pylori associated chronic gastritis, clinical syndromes, precancerous lesions, and pathogenesis of gastric cancer development. World Journal of Gastroenterology. 2014;**20**(18):5461-5473

[10] Malfertheiner P, Megraud F, O'Morain C, Bazzoli F, El-Omar E, Graham D, et al. Current concepts in the management of *Helicobacter pylori* infection: The Maastricht III Consensus Report. Gut. Jun 2007;**56**(6):772-781

[11] Wang J, Xu L, Shi R, Huang X, Li SW, Huang Z, et al. Gastric atrophy and intestinal metaplasia before and after *Helicobacter pylori* eradication: A meta-analysis. Digestion. 2011;**83**(4):253-260

[12] Lahner E, Carabotti M, Annibale B. Treatment of *Helicobacter pylori* infection in atrophic gastritis. World Journal of Gastroenterology. 2018;**24**(22):2373-2380

[13] Shevtsov MA, Smagina LV, Kudriavtceva TA, Petlenko SV, Voronkina IV. Glu-Trp-ONa or its acylated analogue (R-Glu-Trp-ONa) administration enhances the wound healing in the model of chronic skin wounds in rabbits. Drug Design and Developmental Therapy. 2015;**9**:1717-1727

[14] Kasimova AR, Petlenko IS, Bozhkova SA. Dynamics of postsurgical wound local changes and healing rate during the use of alpha-glutamyl-tryptophan in combination therapy of patients with skin and soft-tissue infections. Siberian Scientific Medical Journal. 2020;**40**(5):98-105

[15] Petlenko IS, Egorova TY, Petlenko SV, et al. Experimental study of the specific activity of L-Glutamyl- L-Tryptophan. Modern Problems of Science and Education. 2019;**3**:199

Chapter 3

Helicobacter pylori: A Bacterium Influencing and Causing Most of the Diseases in the Upper Gastrointestinal Tract – An Overview with Respect to Pathogenesis and Treatment Based on Basic Physiology

Helge L. Waldum

Abstract

The discovery that *Helicobacter pylori* was the dominating cause of gastritis is among the most important findings in the last century. It gave rise to the understanding and treatment of serious and common diseases, such as peptic ulcer disease and gastric cancer. The gastric hormone gastrin is involved in the pathogenesis of both duodenal ulcer and gastric cancer, whereas reduction in the defense mechanism (mucus and bicarbonate) by the inflammation itself predisposes to gastric ulcer. The search for carcinogenic *H. pylori* factors has been unsuccessful and based upon the fact that *H. pylori* predispose to gastric cancer only after having induced oxyntic atrophy is an important argument in favor of a central role of gastrin increase secondary to reduced acidity. The only cell with an undisputed gastrin receptor is the enterochromaffin-like cell where gastrin has a trophic effect leading to hyperplasia, neuroendocrine tumor (NET), and long-term carcinoma of diffuse type. *H. pylori* may be eradicated by a combination of antibiotics with a potent inhibitor of acid secretion. *H. pylori* is dependent on acid surrounding to thrive, and therefore anacidity due to complete oxyntic atrophy or profound inhibition of acid secretion by drugs will promote its disappearance.

Keywords: *Helicobacter pylori*, duodenal ulcer, gastric peptic ulcer, gastric cancer, gastrin, enterochromaffin-like cell

1. Introduction

Diseases of the upper gastrointestinal tract, such as peptic ulcer and gastric cancer, were previously very prevalent. Moreover, gastric cancer has high mortality, and

IntechOpen

peptic ulcer was an important disabling disease. With different types of surgical interventions on the regulation of acid secretion, such as removal of the gastrin-producing antrum or cutting of the vagal nerves, the prognosis of severe peptic ulcer disease improved but not seldom with serious postoperative complaints. With the description of the histamine 2(H2) receptor and the development of the first H2 receptor antagonist, cimetidine, by Black and coworkers [1], peptic ulcer disease became available for drug treatment. Later the more efficient inhibitor of acid secretion, omeprazole, was described and found to inhibit the final step in acid secretion, the proton pump (PPI) [2, 3]. Drugs inhibiting gastric acid secretion when dosed sufficiently made virtually every peptic ulcer heal but had to be continued indefinitely to prevent relapses. At the same time period, it was realized that peptic ulcer disease was associated with gastritis [4, 5].

Similarly, gastritis was recognized as a factor in gastric carcinogenesis [6, 7] in the 1950s, while a role of gastric hypoacidity was described the decade before [8, 9]. Gastritis was, thus, established as central in diseases of the upper gastrointestinal tract. The etiology of gastritis was unknown, but based upon distribution, two types of gastritis were described as type A only affecting the oxyntic mucosa and type B affecting the antral mucosa and gradually spreading to the oxyntic mucosa [10]. Thus, there was apparent that gastritis was very important in upper gastrointestinal pathology and that there existed two types of gastritis with presumed different etiology before Marshall and Warren made their description of *H. pylori* (*H. pylori*) [11], which subsequently has been shown to be the major cause of peptic ulcer [12], as well as gastric cancer [13].

2. *H. pylori*

Around nineteen hundred "spirochete" resembling organisms were recognized in the gastric mucosa [14] in gastric tissue taken from stomachs with gastric cancer [15]. Similarly, epidemic gastritis with hypochlorhydria was reported in the fifties [16] and in the late seventies, the occurrence of gastritis leading to hypoacidity was described as to result of contaminated gastric tubes [17]. Likewise, a gastric urease had been described, which subsequently was shown to be of bacterial origin since tetracycline treatment changed gastric juice nitrogen from ammonium to urea [18]. The indications for an infectious agent causing gastritis accumulated during the nearly hundred years period ahead of the culture of the organism now known as *H. pylori* [11] are excellently summarized by Marshall himself [18]. *H. pylori* produces many factors that make the bacterium able to live in the gastric mucus, as well as to induce damage and inflammation in the epithelial cells. The urease is essential for its ability to survive in the highly acidic stomach, whereas the cytotoxin-associated gene A (Gag A) probably is most important in inducing inflammation, damage to the gastric mucosa, and diseases [19].

2.1 Urease

The high production of urease by *H. pylori* is a central trait for thriving in the gastric mucus [20] and is also the basis for the rapid urease test to diagnose gastric infection with *H. pylori* [21]. In the eradication cures of *H. pylori*, potent inhibition of acid secretion is combined with high doses of antibiotics, and it is probable that the reduction in acidity of the mucus contributes to the killing of the bacterium. Potassium-competitive acid blockers (P-CABs) are even more effective than proton pump inhibitors (PPIs) in inhibiting acid secretion. In combination with amoxicillin and clarithromycin, vonoprazan (a P-CAB) induced the same degree of *H. pylori* eradication after one-week therapy as with the same antibiotics at the same doses together with PPIs for 2 weeks [22].

2.2 Blood group antigen binding adhesin A (Bab A)

Urease activity of *H. pylori* is necessary for both establishing and persistence of infection [20]. The initial binding of *H. pylori* to the gastric mucosal cells depends on adhesins. Among them, Bab A has been considered particularly important, although the clinical implications of the different expressions seem marginal [23].

2.3 Cytotoxin-associated gene A (Cag A)

Among the virulence factors in *H. pylori*, Cag A is probably the most important. Cag A gene is part of the cytotoxin-associated gene pathogenicity island (cagPAI), which also contains the bacterial type IV secretion system (T4SS) whereby Cag A enters the gastric mucosal cells [24]. The presence of cagPAI seems to be associated with more severe gastric pathology, including gastric cancer [19], and some polymorphisms may also have a higher risk [25]. After having penetrated the epithelial cell membrane, Cag A is phosphorylated, and phosphorylated Cag A then interacts with different proteins causing damage to the infected cell [19]. However, any direct mechanism for the pathogenetic effect of Cag A or *H. pylori* itself is still missing.

2.4 Vacuolating cytotoxin A (Vac A)

Vac A is a pore-forming protein that binds to some receptors and enters the cell interior by endocytosis [26]. After having entered the cell, Vac A induces large vacuoles [27] and cell death possibly by affecting mitochondrial function [28].

The pathogenetic role of the different factors of *H. pylori* has been discussed in depth in different recent reviews [19, 29], but the exact mechanism for the carcinogenic effect has not been disclosed. Already, in 2000, Graham and Yamaoka wrote a review with the title: Disease-specific *H. pylori* virulence factors: the unfilled promise [30]. They concluded that only the cag pathogenicity island had passed the tests of biological plausibility with respect to increased inflammation. Subsequently, I will describe the course of *H. pylori* infection and afterward return to the question of the pathogenesis of gastric cancer due to *H. pylori*.

2.5 Course of *H. pylori* infection

The symptoms of acute *H. pylori* infection are probably best described by the two known voluntary infections [31, 32]. As early as 3 days after ingestion of *H. pylori* epigastric pains were noticed and mild symptoms persisted for 14 days. Normal gastric acidity before infection was changed to anacidity on day 8 after infection [32]. Interestingly, these two voluntary infections were successful only after giving an inhibitor of gastric acid secretion suggesting that gastric acidity protects to some degree against initial infection. In this context, it shall also be mentioned the outbreak of gastritis due to contamination of the equipment in a study of gastric secretion described in 1979 [17]. The healthy subjects were tested multiple times and developed epigastric symptoms, gastritis, and hypoacidity. In retrospect, this outbreak of hypo-acidic gastritis has been attributed to contamination with *H. pylori*. It should be noticed that also in these subjects *H. pylori* most probably was introduced into the stomach with hypoacidity since the gastric juice was continuously aspirated [33]. What about the role of gastric acidity in real-life initial steps of infection?

It is well-known that *H. pylori* infection occurs mainly in childhood both in developed and developing countries [34, 35]. Although gastric acidity is lower during the first year of life compared with healthy individuals later in life [36], a difference in gastric acidity cannot explain the different susceptibility for *H. pylori* infection in childhood. The habit of small children putting so many things into their mouths may perhaps contribute. The present prevalent use of profound inhibitors of acid secretion in adults seen during the last decades has not resulted in any increased tendency to new *H. pylori* infections in grown-ups, indicating that hypoacidity is not as important for establishing *H. pylori* infection as the two voluntary studies [31, 32] suggested. On the other hand, in those studies acid secretion was inhibited by a histamine blocker, thus only moderate reduction in gastric acidity compared with PPIs. It is possible that profound acid inhibition could reduce the susceptibility for *H. pylori* infection due to a reduction in acidity in gastric mucous. In contrast, PPI treatment has been reported to increase the proximal spread of *H. pylori* gastritis [37] possibly by reducing mucous acidity reflecting that *H. pylori* require some acidity, but not too high acidity as patients with gastrinoma generally have a low frequency of *H. pylori* infection [38].

The mechanism for the initial inhibition of acid secretion is not completely elucidated, but hypoacidity may persist for weeks or even months [17]. After ingestion, *H. pylori* first infects the antral mucosa but after days spreads to the oxyntic mucosa as well [31, 32]. Properties both by *H. pylori* itself, and the inflammation provoked have been implicated [33, 39]. For some reason or the other, the transition from acute to chronic gastritis is accompanied by resolution of the inflammation in the oxyntic mucosa, whereas it persists in the antral mucosa. Concomitant with the healing of the oxyntic mucosa, gastric acidity is normalized [17, 32]. The general belief is that when first infected, *H. pylori* infection will persist until eventual eradication or reaching complete anacidity secondary to atrophic oxyntic atrophy. In some patients, *H. pylori* gastritis remain confined to the antral mucosa for years, whereas in others *H. pylori* and accompanying gastritis early spread in the oral direction. The reason for this difference is not known, but the fact that inhibition of gastric acid secretion promotes the distribution of gastritis orally [40] and may suggest that acidity plays a role [33].

The development of the *H. pylori* gastritis has a dual effect on gastric acid secretion. When the infection is confined to the antral mucosa, gastric acid secretion is increased due to elevated gastrin release [41], whereas gastric acid secretion is impaired when oxyntic gastritis with damage to the parietal cells has occurred. It is probable that the increase in gastrin release, in relation to gastric acidity (inappropriate gastrin release), is due to an effect on gastrin release by NH3 produced by *H. pylori* urease. Studies to examine whether NH3 could be the causative factor for this effect on gastrin release have been ambivalent, but in a careful evaluation of the data related to this question, we concluded that *H. pylori*-induced NH3 was the cause of inappropriate gastrin release and thus hypersecretion of acid [33].

Subsequently, the inflammation in most patients spreads to the oxyntic mucosa. Why some patients are more resistant to oxyntic affection is not known. Similarly, the reason why the oxyntic mucosa is apparently less susceptible to *H. pylori* gastritis than the antral mucosa is also unknown. However, it is thought that higher acidity could play a role. Nevertheless, the oxyntic glands empty their contents into the lumen through transient openings and not by diffusion through the mucous layer. Anyhow, the luminal acidity is slightly higher in the oxyntic area, and this could play a role in the relative resistance. The oxyntic *H. pylori* gastritis starts as superficial gastritis, which gradually affects the deeper layers of the mucosa including the glands finally destroying them and leading to reduced acid production by the disappearance of the parietal cells and other specialized cells, such as the chief cells. All the specialized cells of the oxyntic mucosa are killed during this process except the target cell of gastrin, the enterochromaffin-like (ECL) cell [42]. With time, all the oxyntic mucosa is destroyed leading to anacidity and disappearance of the *H. pylori* infection [43] since the bacterium depends on some acidity in the surroundings to neutralize the NH_3 production caused by the urease. The complete atrophy of the oxyntic mucosa naturally leads to hypergastrinemia [44].

2.6 Consequences of *H. pylori* infection

2.6.1 Gastritis

The acute infection causes acute gastritis, which subsides within a week or two. Chronic uncomplicated phase of gastritis does not cause any symptoms, which is exemplified by the previous belief that gastritis could be regarded as a normal phenomenon of older age. However, chronic *H. pylori* gastritis is complicated with many serious upper gastrointestinal diseases; in fact, most of the diseases in the upper gastrointestinal tract are influenced or caused by this infection.

2.6.2 Peptic ulcer disease

Peptic ulcer disease consists of two subgroups: duodenal and gastric ulcers. At both locations, the ulcer is caused by the digestion of the mucosa by the acidic and proteolytic gastric juice. In duodenal ulcer, the aggressive forces are increased as shown by the increased acid secretion [45], whereas in gastric ulcers, a reduction in defense (bicarbonate and mucous production by superficial cells) is probably the mechanism. *H. pylori* gastritis has been shown to inhibit mucin synthesis [46]. Generally, the more oral a gastric ulcer is localized, the lower is the capacity to produce acid [45]. Also, reflux oesophagitis is ultimately due to the erosive activity of gastric juice. The roles of acid versus pepsin in tissue damage in all these conditions are difficult to differentiate since the regulations of pepsinogen, and acid secretions in many ways are similar. Furthermore, acid is required for the autocatalytic activation of pepsinogen into the active form pepsin [47]. The most important factor in the pathogenesis of reflux oesophagitis is insufficiency of the functional gastro-esophageal valve, whereas *H. pylori* is the dominating cause of both duodenal and gastric ulcers. *H. pylori* gastritis influences the risk and severity of gastro-esophageal reflux through the reduction of gastric acid secretion due to oxyntic atrophy [33].

2.6.3 Duodenal ulcer

Duodenal ulcer has for long been known to be associated with increased gastric acid secretion [45]. Concomitant with the description that *H. pylori* was the dominating cause of gastritis, it was also shown that most patients with peptic ulcer, being duodenal or gastric, also were infected [11]. Initially, it was thought that duodenal ulcers occurred at islands of gastric metaplasia in the duodenum. This has not been substantiated [48, 49], and the focus has been directed toward the elevation of gastric acid secretion. It was detected that patients with antral gastritis had a slight elevation of gastrin in the blood causing an increase in gastric acid secretion [33, 41]. The pathogenesis of duodenal ulcer is, thus, most likely the increase in gastric acid secretion due to *H. pylori* infection of the antrum. An increase in gastric acid secretion is alone sufficient to induce peptic ulcer as shown in non-infected patients with gastrinoma [38]. Moreover, the lower frequency of *H. pylori* in gastrinoma patients compared with age-matched controls suggests that high acidity can eradicate *H. pylori* since infection with *H. pylori* most often occurs in childhood, and gastrinoma seldom manifests itself before adulthood [33]. *H. pylori* eradication reduces gastrin and gastric acid secretion and prevents new ulcers, in other words, cures duodenal ulcer disease [41, 50].

2.6.4 Gastric peptic ulcer

In gastric peptic ulcers, it is the defense mechanisms (bicarbonate and mucous) that are reduced and not an increase in aggressive factors that cause the ulcers. The decline in the defense factors is caused by *H. pylori* gastritis [46] in most instances but may also be due to other factors with intake of nonsteroidal anti-inflammatory drugs (NSAIDs) as the most important one. The effect of NSAIDs on the gastric mucosa is related to their ability to inhibit prostaglandin synthesis [51]. Prostaglandin treatment may prevent development or heal gastric ulcers [52]. The distribution between *H. pylori* and NSAIDs use as the cause of peptic gastric ulcer depends on the time for the study, the age of the patients, as well as their country, because the prevalence of *H. pylori* in many populations is rapidly declining and shows great variability between countries. Of course, whenever *H. pylori* is found in a patient with upper gastrointestinal disease, it should be eradicated. The treatment of NSAID- induced gastric ulcers is termination of NSAID use when possible, or otherwise add an inhibitor of gastric acid secretion or possibly a prostaglandin analog.

2.6.5 Gastro-esophageal reflux disease

Patients with duodenal ulcer have increased gastric acid secretion, which can induce reflux symptoms as exemplified in patients with gastrinoma [53]. Such symptoms may occur in patients with duodenal ulcer, but the increase in gastric acid secretion due to antral *H. pylori* gastritis seldom leads to reflux oesophagitis, possibly due to maintained regulation of gastrin release, and thus only a marginal increase in gastrin. On the other hand, *H. pylori* gastritis leading to oxyntic atrophy may reduce the occurrence of gastrointestinal reflux due to impaired gastric acid secretion [54]. Thus, *H. pylori* may induce gastro-esophageal symptoms or at another phase of gastritis reduce such symptoms. Generally, it may be stated that *H. pylori* does not play any central role in gastro-esophageal reflux disease.

2.6.6 Gastric cancer

An old slogan was “no acid, no peptic ulcer.” Similarly, with some limitations, it may be said: “no gastritis, no gastric cancer” [6]. After the recognition that *H. pylori* was the major cause of gastritis [11], it was logical that *H. pylori* also was an important contributor to gastric cancer [13]. This induced a search for the carcinogenic factor in *H. pylori*, the first bacterium to be accepted to be carcinogenic. Despite intense work by many groups for many years, the mechanism has not been disclosed leading to the paper containing: "unfulfilled promise" in the title [30]. However, major progress was done by the recognition that *H. pylori* did not cause gastric cancer before having induced oxyntic atrophy [55]. Moreover, even after the disappearance of *H. pylori* either due to eradication therapy or complete oxyntic atrophy leading to anacidity, patients having been infected for years have an increased risk for gastric cancer for decades after the loss of the bacterium [56]. Also, when the infection was confined to the antral mucosa, the patients were not predisposed to gastric cancer. On the contrary, patients with a duodenal ulcer, which has mainly antral gastritis, have lower cancer risk than controls [57]. Altogether, these data do not support a direct carcinogen effect of *H. pylori*. In any way, carcinogenesis is connected to induced gastritis in the oxyntic mucosa. Among the *H. pylori* factors, Cag A seems to be the most important in the pathogenesis of gastritis, although its direct role in gastric carcinogenesis beyond driving the inflammation is still not disclosed [19]. The *H. pylori* infection goes through stages from superficial to atrophic gastritis, and the latter may be complicated by intestinal metaplasia [58]. Intestinal metaplasia has been regarded as a very important step and according to Correa [59], being a precursor to gastric cancer of the intestinal type (Lauren [60]). However, the importance of intestinal metaplasia in carcinogenesis has been questioned [61, 62], and intestinal metaplasia may only be a marker of long-standing oxyntic atrophy [63]. It, thus, seems that atrophic gastritis is central in gastric carcinogenesis, a condition that leads to reduced killing of swallowed micro-organisms, as well as hypergastrinemia. If changes in microbiological milieu secondary to impaired gastric acid secretion are the mechanism, it is peculiar that patients with autoimmune gastritis do develop cancers only in the oxyntic mucosa, and not the whole stomach [64]. Therefore, hypergastrinemia may be the factor mediating the cancers induced by *H. pylori* [63]. This concept is compatible with no increase or lower incidence of gastric cancers in patients with duodenal ulcers [57], as well as the continuous predisposition decades after eradication of the bacterium [56]. This view has implications for the treatment with *H. pylori* eradication in those still being infected, and the use of a gastrin analog such as netazepide [65] in those having oxyntic atrophy and hypergastrinemia but having lost the bacterium.

H. pylori gastritis also predisposes to gastric lymphoma so-called mucosa-associated lymphoid tumor (MALT). In contrast to gastric carcinomas, these tumors develop because of the continuous and chronic inflammation itself and are independent of gastric atrophy [66]. Many of the gastric MALT-lymphomas associated with *H. pylori* may be cured by *H. pylori* eradication [67].

2.6.7 H. pylori *eradication: When and how*

H. pylori is an important cause of serious diseases. The eradication of *H. pylori* in peptic ulcer diseases cures the diseases, which previously were rather frequent and could have grave consequences. Gastric cancer was among the most common cancers and had and still has a high mortality. During the last fifty years, there has been a remarkable decline in occurrence of gastric cancer [68], most probably due to a decline in infection with *H. pylori*, especially in the Western world. However, still, a proportion of the population is infected, and in non-Western countries, the percentage infected is even today high [69]. The spontaneous reduction in infection rate seen during the last decades is attributed to improved hygienic conditions. Most of the infections occur in childhood and even above the age of five years, reinfection is seldom [70]. After infection, chronic gastritis develops spreading slowly to include the oxyntic mucosa and gradually destroying the specialized cells leading to atrophy.

Atrophy usually precedes development of intestinal metaplasia [71]. Uemura and coworkers showed that *H. pylori* infection predisposed to gastric cancer first after having induced oxyntic atrophy [55], and a separate role of intestinal metaplasia in gastric carcinogenesis as suggested by Correa [59] is not ambiguously accepted [61, 62]. Alternatively, intestinal metaplasia could just be a consequence of long-standing atrophy [63]. Anyhow, to prevent common and serious diseases, such as peptic ulcer disease and gastric cancer, *H. pylori* should be eradicated before irreversible atrophic gastritis has developed. Since *H. pylori* infection occurs in childhood and the actual diseases, as well as atrophic gastritis seldom, occurs in young people, the natural conclusion is that all should be tested for *H. pylori* infection around the age of twenty years, and those positive should have *H. pylori* eradicated at that age. Eradication of *H. pylori* has traditionally been achieved by a combination of two or more antibiotics and rather early together with an inhibitor of acid secretion. Bismuth salts were among the first to show efficacy in *H. pylori* eradication [72]. Antibiotic resistance has been a problem in the eradication of *H. pylori* [73]. The initial argument for adding an inhibitor of acid secretion was to prevent destruction of the antibiotics in the stomach, thus prolonging their local effect. To achieve acceptable *H. pylori* eradication, cures of two weeks duration were most often required. Recently, the potassium-competitive acid blocker (P-CAB) vonoprazan in combination with amoxicillin, and clarithromycin for 1 week was as efficient in eradicating *H. pylori* compared to the same antibiotics in combination with PPIs for 2 weeks [22], indicating that even more complete acid inhibition further improved the efficacy of the treatment cure. In other words, the more efficient inhibition of gastric acid secretion, the more likely *H. pylori* will not survive reflecting the self-toxicity by NH3 produced by its urease. It is conceivable that high doses of P-CABs will totally remove gastric acidity, and thus be suitable for *H. pylori* eradication alone. The reported bactericide effect on *H. pylori* by high doses of PPIs most probably is caused by the dependence of some acidity in the surrounding of *H. pylori* [74]. Of course, such treatment will naturally induce marked hypergastrinemia, which could make harm even during a short period but could be prevented by a gastrin antagonist. Marked oxyntic atrophy after *H. pylori* eradication and termination of inflammation nevertheless predisposes to gastric cancer, which probably is caused by the corresponding hypergastrinemia. Thus, such patients will most likely also profit from treatment with a gastrin antagonist [75].

3. Conclusion

The description of *H. pylori* as the main cause of gastritis leading to peptic ulcer disease, and gastric cancer is among the most important achievement in medicine in the last century. This allows prevention of such important diseases and opens up for an understanding of new mechanisms in diseases, including cancer. Together with the hormone gastrin, *H. pylori* may explain most aspects of diseases of the upper gastrointestinal tract. It is probable that a similar cause/mechanism also is found in other organs, but it is not surprising that it is first disclosed in the stomach, an organ ideal for studying biological mechanisms.

Conflict of interest

The authors declare no conflict of interest.

Author details

Helge L. Waldum
Faculty of Medicine and Health Sciences, Department of Clinical and Molecular Medicine, Norwegian University of Science and Technology, Trondheim, Norway

*Address all correspondence to: helge.waldum@ntnu.no

References

[1] Black JW, Duncan WA, Durant CJ, Ganellin CR, Parsons EM. Definition and antagonism of histamine H 2 - receptors. Nature. 1972;**236**:385-390. DOI: 10.1038/236385a0

[2] Sachs G, Chang HH, Rabon E, Schackman R, Lewin M, Saccomani G. A nonelectrogenic H+ pump in plasma membranes of hog stomach. The Journal of Biological Chemistry. 1976;**251**:7690-7698

[3] Sachs G, Wallmark B. Biological basis of omeprazole therapy. Journal of Gastroenterology and Hepatology. 1989;**4**(Suppl. 2):7-18

[4] Gear MW, Truelove SC, Whitehead R. Gastric ulcer and gastritis. Gut. 1971;**12**:639-645. DOI: 10.1136/gut.12.8.639

[5] Tatsuta M, Iishi H, Okuda S. Location of peptic ulcers in relation to antral and fundal gastritis by chromoendoscopic follow-up examinations. Digestive Diseases and Sciences. 1986;**31**:7-11. DOI: 10.1007/bf01347902

[6] Morson BC. Intestinal metaplasia of the gastric mucosa. British Journal of Cancer. 1955;**9**:365-376. DOI: 10.1038/bjc.1955.35

[7] Siurala M, Seppala K. Atrophic gastritis as a possible precursor of gastric carcinoma and pernicious anemia. Results of follow-up examinations. Acta Medica Scandinavica. 1960;**166**:455-474

[8] Comfort MW, Kelsey MP, Berkson J. Gastric acidity before and after the development of carcinoma of the stomach. Collected Papers of the Mayo Clinic and the Mayo Foundation. 1946;**38**:24-30

[9] Chitre RG, Samant VG. Anacidity in gastric cancer. The Indian Medical Gazette. 1944;**79**:472-475

[10] Strickland RG. Type a and B atrophic gastritis. Journal of Clinical Gastroenterology. 1983;**5**:477-478. DOI: 10.1097/00004836-198310000-00023

[11] Marshall BJ, Warren JR. Unidentified curved bacilli in the stomach of patients with gastritis and peptic ulceration. Lancet. 1984;**1**:1311-1315

[12] Marshall BJ. Helicobacter pylori in peptic ulcer: Have Koch's postulates been fulfilled? Annals of Medicine. 1995;**27**:565-568. DOI: 10.3109/07853899509002470

[13] Parsonnet J, Friedman GD, Vandersteen DP, Chang Y, Vogelman JH, Orentreich N, et al. Helicobacter pylori infection and the risk of gastric carcinoma. The New England Journal of Medicine. 1991;**325**:1127-1131. DOI: 10.1056/nejm199110173251603

[14] Bizzozero G. Ueber die schlauchformigen drusen des magendarmkanals und die bezienhungen ihres epithels zu dem oberflachenepithel der schleimhaut. Arch Mikr Anat. 1893;**42**:82

[15] Krienitz W. Ueber das Auftreten von Spirochaeten verschiedener Form in Mageninhalt bei Carcinoma ventriculi. DtschMed Wochenschr. 1906;**32**:872

[16] Hirschowitz BI, London JA, Pollard HM, Streeten DH. A steroid-induced gastric ulcer. Lancet (London, England). 1956;**271**:1081-1083. DOI: 10.1016/s0140-6736(56)90214-8

[17] Ramsey EJ, Carey KV, Peterson WL, Jackson JJ, Murphy FK, Read NW, et al. Epidemic gastritis with hypochlorhydria. Gastroenterology. 1979;**76**:1449-1457

[18] Marshall BJ. One hundred years of discovery and rediscovery of Herlicobacter pylori and its association with peptic ulcer disease. In: HLT M, MG, Hazell SL, editors. Helicobacter pylori: Physiology and Genetics. Washington (DC): ASM Press; 2001

[19] Ansari S, Yamaoka Y. Helicobacter pylori virulence factor Cytotoxin-associated gene a (CagA)-mediated gastric pathogenicity. International Journal of Molecular Sciences. 2020;**21**:7430. DOI: 10.3390/ijms21197430

[20] Debowski AW, Walton SM, Chua EG, Tay AC, Liao T, Lamichhane B, et al. Helicobacter pylori gene silencing in vivo demonstrates urease is essential for chronic infection. PLoS Pathogens. 2017;**13**:e1006464. DOI: 10.1371/journal.ppat.1006464

[21] Marshall BJ, Warren JR, Francis GJ, Langton SR, Goodwin CS, Blincow ED. Rapid urease test in the management of Campylobacter pyloridis-associated gastritis. The American Journal of Gastroenterology. 1987;**82**:200-210

[22] Ang D, Koo SH, Chan YH, Tan TY, Soon GH, Tan CK, et al. Clinical trial: Seven-day vonoprazan- versus 14-day proton pump inhibitor-based triple therapy for first-line Helicobacter pylori eradication. Alimentary Pharmacology & Therapeutics. 2022;**56**:436-449. DOI: 10.1111/apt.17070

[23] Fujimoto S, Olaniyi Ojo O, Arnqvist A, Wu JY, Odenbreit S, Haas R, et al. Helicobacter pylori BabA expression, gastric mucosal injury, and clinical outcome. Clinical Gastroenterology and Hepatology. 2007;**5**:49-58. DOI: 10.1016/j.cgh.2006.09.015

[24] Backert S, Tegtmeyer N, Fischer W. Composition, structure and function of the Helicobacter pylori cag pathogenicity island encoded type IV secretion system. Future Microbiology. 2015;**10**:955-965. DOI: 10.2217/fmb.15.32

[25] CanzianF, RizzatoC, ObazeeO, SteinA, Flores-Luna L, Camorlinga-Ponce M, et al. Genetic polymorphisms in the cag pathogenicity island of Helicobacter pylori and risk of stomach cancer and high-grade premalignant gastric lesions. International Journal of Cancer. 2020;**147**:2437-2445. DOI: 10.1002/ijc.33032

[26] Gauthier NC, Monzo P, Kaddai V, Doye A, Ricci V, Boquet P. Helicobacter pylori VacA cytotoxin: A probe for a clathrin-independent and Cdc42-dependent pinocytic pathway routed to late endosomes. Molecular Biology of the Cell. 2005;**16**:4852-4866. DOI: 10.1091/mbc.e05-05-0398

[27] Utsch C, Haas R. VacA's induction of VacA-containing vacuoles (VCVs) and their immunomodulatory activities on human T cells. Toxins (Basel). 2016;**8**:190. DOI: 10.3390/toxins8060190

[28] Yamasaki E, Wada A, Kumatori A, Nakagawa I, Funao J, Nakayama M, et al. Helicobacter pylori vacuolating cytotoxin induces activation of the proapoptotic proteins Bax and Bak, leading to cytochrome c release and cell death, independent of vacuolation. The Journal of Biological Chemistry. 2006;**281**:11250-11259. DOI: 10.1074/jbc.M509404200

[29] Alexander SM, Retnakumar RJ, Chouhan D, Devi TNB, Dharmaseelan S, Devadas K, et al. Helicobacter pylori in human stomach: The inconsistencies in clinical outcomes and the probable causes. Frontiers in Microbiology. 2021;**12**:713955. DOI: 10.3389/fmicb.2021.713955

[30] Graham DY, Yamaoka Y. Disease-specific Helicobacter pylori virulence

factors: The unfulfilled promise. Helicobacter. 2000;**5**(Suppl. 1):S3-S9; discussion S27-31. DOI: 10.1046/j.1523-5378.2000.0050s1003.x

[31] Marshall BJ, Armstrong JA, McGechie DB, Glancy RJ. Attempt to fulfil Koch's postulates for pyloric Campylobacter. The Medical Journal of Australia. 1985;**142**:436-439. DOI: 10.5694/j.1326-5377.1985.tb113443.x

[32] Morris A, Nicholson G. Ingestion of Campylobacter pyloridis causes gastritis and raised fasting gastric pH. The American Journal of Gastroenterology. 1987;**82**:192-199

[33] Waldum HL, Kleveland PM, Sordal OF. Helicobacter pylori and gastric acid: An intimate and reciprocal relationship. Therapeutic Advances in Gastroenterology. 2016;**9**:836-844. DOI: 10.1177/1756283x16663395

[34] Thomas JE, Dale A, Harding M, Coward WA, Cole TJ, Weaver LT. Helicobacter pylori colonization in early life. Pediatric Research. 1999;**45**:218-223. DOI: 10.1203/00006450-199902000-00010

[35] Lindkvist P, Asrat D, Nilsson I, Tsega E, Olsson GL, Wretlind B, et al. Age at acquisition of Helicobacter pylori infection: Comparison of a high and a low prevalence country. Scandinavian Journal of Infectious Diseases. 1996;**28**:181-184. DOI: 10.3109/00365549609049072

[36] Becker M, Fritsch WP, Hausamen TU, Rotthauwe HW. Serum-gastrin levels and gastric-acid secretion in infants (author's transl). Deutsche Medizinische Wochenschrift. 1976;**101**:1800-1805. DOI: 10.1055/s-0028-1104342

[37] Kuipers EJ, Lee A, Klinkenberg-Knol EC, Meuwissen SG. Review article: The development of atrophic gastritis--Helicobacter pylori and the effects of acid suppressive therapy. Alimentary Pharmacology & Therapeutics. 1995;**9**:331-340. DOI: 10.1111/j.1365-2036.1995.tb00391.x

[38] Weber HC, Venzon DJ, Jensen RT, Metz DC. Studies on the interrelation between Zollinger-Ellison syndrome, Helicobacter pylori, and proton pump inhibitor therapy. Gastroenterology. 1997;**112**:84-91. DOI: 10.1016/s0016-5085(97)70222-1

[39] Calam J. Pathogenic mechanisms. Baillière's Clinical Gastroenterology. 1995;**9**:487-506. DOI: 10.1016/0950-3528(95)90044-6

[40] Logan RP, Walker MM, Misiewicz JJ, Gummett PA, Karim QN, Baron JH. Changes in the intragastric distribution of Helicobacter pylori during treatment with omeprazole. Gut. 1995;**36**:12-16. DOI: 10.1136/gut.36.1.12

[41] Levi S, Beardshall K, Haddad G, Playford R, Ghosh P, Calam J. Campylobacter pylori and duodenal ulcers: The gastrin link. Lancet. 1989;**1**:1167-1168. DOI: 10.1016/s0140-6736(89)92752-9

[42] Waldum HL, Sørdal ØF, Mjønes PG. The Enterochromaffin-like [ECL] cell-central in gastric physiology and pathology. International Journal of Molecular Sciences. 2019;**20**:5203. DOI: 10.3390/ijms20102444

[43] Karnes WE Jr, Samloff IM, Siurala M, Kekki M, Sipponen P, Kim SW, et al. Positive serum antibody and negative tissue staining for Helicobacter pylori in subjects with atrophic body gastritis. Gastroenterology. 1991;**101**:167-174. DOI: 10.1016/0016-5085(91)90474-y

[44] Trudeau WL, McGuigan JE. Relations between serum gastrin levels

and rates of gastric hydrochloric acid secretion. The New England Journal of Medicine. 1971;**284**:408-412. DOI: 10.1056/nejm197102252840803

[45] Wormsley KG, Grossman MI. Maximal histalog test in control subjects and patients with peptic ulcer. Gut. 1965;**6**:427-435. DOI: 10.1136/gut.6.5.427

[46] Byrd JC, Yunker CK, Xu QS, Sternberg LR, Bresalier RS. Inhibition of gastric mucin synthesis by Helicobacter pylori. Gastroenterology. 2000;**118**:1072-1079. DOI: 10.1016/s0016-5085(00)70360-x

[47] Herriott RM. Pepsinogen and pepsin. The Journal of General Physiology. 1962;**45**((4)Pt 2):57-76

[48] Csendes A, Smok G, Burdiles P, Blanco C, Rodas J. Presence of Helicobacter pylori in the duodenum, antrum, and fundus in control subjects and patients with duodenal ulcer, gastric ulcer, gastritis, or erosive duodenitis. Histological analysis of 357 subjects. Revista Médica de Chile. 1995;**123**:177-184

[49] Genta RM, Kinsey RS, Singhal A, Suterwala S. Gastric foveolar metaplasia and gastric heterotopia in the duodenum: no evidence of an etiologic role for Helicobacter pylori. Human Pathology. 2010;**41**:1593-1600. DOI: 10.1016/j.humpath.2010.04.010

[50] Rauws EA, Tytgat GN. Cure of duodenal ulcer associated with eradication of Helicobacter pylori. Lancet. 1990;**335**:1233-1235. DOI: 10.1016/0140-6736(90)91301-p

[51] Laine L, Takeuchi K, Tarnawski A. Gastric mucosal defense and cytoprotection: Bench to bedside. Gastroenterology. 2008;**135**:41-60. DOI: 10.1053/j.gastro.2008.05.030

[52] Takeuchi K, Amagase K. Roles of cyclooxygenase, prostaglandin E2 and EP receptors in mucosal protection and ulcer healing in the gastrointestinal tract. Current Pharmaceutical Design. 2018;**24**:2002-2011. DOI: 10.2174/1381612824666180629111227

[53] Rossi RE, Elvevi A, Citterio D, Coppa J, Invernizzi P, Mazzaferro V, et al. Gastrinoma and Zollinger Ellison syndrome: A roadmap for the management between new and old therapies. World Journal of Gastroenterology. 2021;**27**:5890-5907. DOI: 10.3748/wjg.v27.i35.5890

[54] Han YM, Chung SJ, Yoo S, Yang JI, Choi JM, Lee J, et al. Inverse correlation between gastroesophageal reflux disease and atrophic gastritis assessed by endoscopy and serology. World Journal of Gastroenterology. 2022;**28**:853-867. DOI: 10.3748/wjg.v28.i8.853

[55] Uemura N, Okamoto S, Yamamoto S, Matsumura N, Yamaguchi S, Yamakido M, et al. Helicobacter pylori infection and the development of gastric cancer. The New England Journal of Medicine. 2001;**345**:784-789. DOI: 10.1056/NEJMoa001999

[56] Take S, Mizuno M, Ishiki K, Kusumoto C, Imada T, Hamada F, et al. Risk of gastric cancer in the second decade of follow-up after Helicobacter pylori eradication. Journal of Gastroenterology. 2020;**55**:281-288. DOI: 10.1007/s00535-019-01639-w

[57] Hansson LE, Nyrén O, Hsing AW, Bergström R, Josefsson S, Chow WH, et al. The risk of stomach cancer in patients with gastric or duodenal ulcer disease. The New England Journal of Medicine. 1996;**335**:242-249. DOI: 10.1056/nejm199607253350404

[58] El-Zimaity HM. Gastric atrophy, diagnosing and staging. World Journal

of Gastroenterology. 2006;**12**:5757-5762. DOI: 10.3748/wjg.v12.i36.5757

[59] Correa P. Human gastric carcinogenesis: A multistep and multifactorial process--first American Cancer Society award lecture on Cancer epidemiology and prevention. Cancer Research. 1992;**52**:6735-6740

[60] Lauren P. The two histological main types of gastric carcinoma: Diffuse and so-called intestinal-type carcinoma. An attemt at a histo-clinical classification. Acta Pathologica et Microbiologica Scandinavica. 1965;**64**:31-49

[61] Kinoshita H, Hayakawa Y, Koike K. Metaplasia in the stomach-precursor of gastric Cancer? International Journal of Molecular Sciences. 2017;**18**. DOI: 10.3390/ijms18102063

[62] Graham DY, Zou WY. Guilt by association: Intestinal metaplasia does not progress to gastric cancer. Current Opinion in Gastroenterology. 2018;**34**:458-464. DOI: 10.1097/mog.0000000000000472

[63] Waldum HL, Hauso O, Sordal OF, Fossmark R. Gastrin may mediate the carcinogenic effect of Helicobacter pylori infection of the stomach. Digestive Diseases and Sciences. 2015;**60**:1522-1527. DOI: 10.1007/s10620-014-3468-9

[64] Zamcheck N, Grable E, Ley A, Norman L. Occurrence of gastric cancer among patients with pernicious anemia at the Boston City Hospital. The New England Journal of Medicine. 1955;**252**:1103-1110. DOI: 10.1056/nejm195506302522601

[65] Fossmark R, Sørdal Ø, Jianu CS, Qvigstad G, Nordrum IS, Boyce M, et al. Treatment of gastric carcinoids type 1 with the gastrin receptor antagonist netazepide (YF476) results in regression of tumours and normalisation of serum chromogranin a. Alimentary Pharmacology & Therapeutics. 2012;**36**:1067-1075. DOI: 10.1111/apt.12090

[66] Ishikura N, Usui Y, Ito H, Kasugai Y, Oze I, Kato S, et al. Helicobacter pylori (HP) infection alone, but not HP-induced atrophic gastritis, increases the risk of gastric lymphoma: A case-control study in Japan. Annals of Hematology. 2019;**98**:1981-1987. DOI: 10.1007/s00277-019-03721-y

[67] Matysiak-Budnik T, Jamet P, Ruskoné-Fourmestraux A, de Mascarel A, Velten M, Maynadié M, et al. Gastric MALT lymphoma in a population-based study in France: Clinical features, treatments and survival. Alimentary Pharmacology & Therapeutics. 2019;**50**:654-663. DOI: 10.1111/apt.15409

[68] Bray F, Ferlay J, Soerjomataram I, Siegel RL, Torre LA, Jemal A. Global cancer statistics 2018: GLOBOCAN estimates of incidence and mortality worldwide for 36 cancers in 185 countries. CA: a Cancer Journal for Clinicians. 2018;**68**:394-424. DOI: 10.3322/caac.21492

[69] Kotilea K, Bontems P, Touati E. Epidemiology, diagnosis and risk factors of Helicobacter pylori infection. Advances in Experimental Medicine and Biology. 2019;**1149**:17-33. DOI: 10.1007/5584_2019_357

[70] Rowland M, Kumar D, Daly L, O'Connor P, Vaughan D, Drumm B. Low rates of Helicobacter pylori reinfection in children. Gastroenterology. 1999;**117**:336-341. DOI: 10.1053/gast.1999.0029900336

[71] Park YH, Kim N. Review of atrophic gastritis and intestinal metaplasia as a premalignant lesion of gastric

cancer. Journal of Cancer Prevention. 2015;**20**:25-40. DOI: 10.15430/jcp.2015.20.1.25

[72] De Giacomo C, Fiocca R, Villani L, Lisato L, Licardi G, Diegoli N, et al. Helicobacter pylori infection and chronic gastritis: Clinical, serological, and histologic correlations in children treated with amoxicillin and colloidal bismuth subcitrate. Journal of Pediatric Gastroenterology and Nutrition. 1990;**11**:310-316

[73] Alarcón T, Domingo D, López-Brea M. Antibiotic resistance problems with Helicobacter pylori. International Journal of Antimicrobial Agents. 1999;**12**:19-26. DOI: 10.1016/s0924-8579(99)00051-5

[74] Mégraud F. Adjuvant therapy for Helicobacter pylori eradication: Role of lansoprazole shown in vitro. Journal of Clinical Gastroenterology. 1995;**20**(Suppl. 1):S24-S27

[75] Waldum H, Mjønes P. Towards understanding of gastric Cancer based upon physiological role of gastrin and ECL cells. Cancers (Basel). 2020;**12**:3477. DOI: 10.3390/cancers12113477

Section 2

The Role of *Helicobacter pylori* Infection in the Development of Extradigestive Diseases

Chapter 4

Extra Digestive Disease and *Helicobacter pylori* Infection

Mihaela-Flavia Avram, Daniela Cornelia Lazăr and Sorin Olariu

Abstract

Helicobacter pylori infection has been associated with gastric pathology and gastric oncogenesis for many years, but its extra-digestive implications are less known. This chapter aims to provide up-to-date information on its potential role in neurological disease (Alzheimer's disease, stroke, multiple sclerosis, Parkinson's disease), dermatological disease (urticaria, rosacea, psoriasis), ophthalmological disease (glaucoma, chorioretinitis, blepharitis), hematologic disease (anemia, thrombocytopenia, neutropenia), as well as cardio-vascular disease (myocardial infarction, coronary atherosclerosis, hypertension), COVID-19, and metabolic pathology (diabetes mellitus, metabolic syndrome). For each group of diseases, a short description will be presented as well as information from published research. It will provide the reader with a global insight into the role of *Helicobacter pylori* in different pathologies.

Keywords: *Helicobacter pylori*, extra-digestive disease, neurological pathology, dermatological disease, ophthalmological disease, hematologic disease, atherosclerosis, metabolic disease, COVID-19

1. Introduction

Helicobacter pylori (HP) is a gram-negative spiral bacillus discovered by Barry Marshall and Robin Warren in 1982. They isolated it in patients with chronic gastritis or gastro-duodenal ulcers, proving its importance as an etiologic factor for these conditions. The two pathologists received a Nobel Prize award for this discovery. In 1994, the World Health Organization recognized HP to be a group 1 gastric cancer carcinogen.

After discovering the multiple implications of HP in gastric pathology, the medical scientific community started to see associations between HP pylori and several extra-gastric diseases. As early as 1994 a relationship between HP infection and coronary heart disease was found in a pilot study on 111 male patients [1]. These results were the starting point of intense scientific efforts to elucidate the mechanisms through which HP contributes to atherosclerosis.

Many other diseases and syndromes and their possible association with HP started to be studied. Pathogenic mechanisms through which HP contributed to certain diseases were discovered. The next step was, naturally, to see if HP eradication improved the outcome of certain diseases or if it lowered the risk of developing certain medical conditions.

The current chapter offers an overview of HP's association with several types of extra digestive diseases. It offers information on its pathogenic role and possible pathogenic mechanisms as well as the potential influence of eradication treatment upon the overall outcome. It covers various diseases (neurological, dermatological, ophthalmic, metabolic, cardiologic, and hematologic) and also discusses the influence of HP infection in COVID-19 patients.

There is a growing number of extra-digestive diseases that are studied in association with HP, and new mechanisms are discovered. This chapter includes only the seven most studied disease categories in relation to HP infection, with the intention of emphasizing the relationship between HP and different extra digestive disorders in this paper, which will enhance the comprehension of HP pathogenic mechanisms, improve clinical prognosis, and guide treatment.

2. Neurological diseases

As HP does not penetrate the central nervous system (CNS), it has been suggested that systemic immunological alterations caused by HP infection may play roles in neurological diseases.

Infection with HP has been demonstrated to induce regulatory T cells (Tregs), which can block adaptive immune responses, resulting in extra-gastric disease regulation [2, 3]. Multiple sclerosis, an inflammatory demyelinating disease of the CNS, has been linked to autoimmune T and B cell responses against CNS antigens; hence, the reduced prevalence of MS in HP-infected patients may be attributable to an increase in Tregs [3, 4].

By stimulating innate immunity, HP infection may contribute to the etiology of CNS disorders. Pro-inflammatory cytokines such as interleukin IL-1, IL-6, and tumor necrosis factor, as well as C-reactive protein, have been found to be elevated in patients with HP [5, 6]. Furthermore, individuals with Parkinson's and Alzheimer's disease had a greater incidence of HP infection compared to controls [7, 8]. Activation of brain resident innate cells, particularly microglia, is a common feature of CNS pathology in both Parkinson's disease and Alzheimer's disease [7].

Alzheimer's disease is one of the most frequent forms of dementia. It causes a progressive decline in cognitive functions. It has a great impact on patients, their families as well as the whole society, as these patients soon require continuous care for long periods of time. Its cause is not well established and no curative treatment is found up to date [9]. HP infection in these patients proved to increase inflammation and negatively impact the cognitive status, patients with HP scored lower mini-mental state examination score [10]. Another study showed a poorer outcome in verbal memory tests in patients HP positive, compared with HP-negative Alzheimer patients [11]. Eradicating HP in these patients has not been proven to be a treatment for Alzheimer's, but there is data indicating that HP treatment improved survival [12].

Ischemic *stroke* is the result of intracranial atherosclerosis. There are recognized risk factors for this condition: age, type 2 diabetes, arterial hypertension, and metabolic syndrome, but these cannot explain all the cases of stroke, so other causes have to be investigated [13]. As chronic inflammation is present in the process of plaque formation, chronic infections need to be investigated as potential risk factors. Several studies showed a correlation between HP and stroke. Positive anti-HP IgG, C-urea breath test, and antiCag-A were significantly associated with a higher risk of stroke [14]. The association is even more evident in women less than 60 years old [15].

Multiple sclerosis is a chronic demyelinating disease of the central nervous system. Its cause is not discovered, but environmental factors are studied in the hope of finding its pathogenesis. Studies have surprisingly shown that HP is less common in patients with multiple sclerosis compared to patients with other neurological pathologies, as well as compared to controls [16, 17]. Experimental studies on mice showed that HP plays a beneficial role in reducing the severity of multiple sclerosis symptoms, possibly providing protection against demyelination [18]. These findings constitute a new direction in the study of the disease.

Parkinson's disease is a degenerative disease affecting the cells in the substantia nigra, which lead to the progressive loss of dopaminergic neurons. Early studies already showed a correlation between HP and this disease, patients with Parkinson's disease having a three times higher risk of testing positive for HP compared to controls [19].

HP infection seems to interfere with the treatment of Parkinson's disease, possibly due to the damage caused by the infection on the mucosa of the duodenum., This leads to an impaired absorption of L-dopa medicine in these patients with the need to increase treatment doses. HP treatment improves patients' response to L-dopa [20]. Eradicating HP proved to improve motor fluctuations and increase the daily 'on' time in advanced Parkinson patients, but no significant improvement in the quality of life was noted [21]. Based on numerous studies, in these patients, HP testing and evaluating the possibility of its eradication when present, seem to play a considerable role in improving treatment outcomes.

3. Dermatological diseases

Urticaria is a common skin disease characterized by edematous, erythematous, itching skin lesions that regress spontaneously within 24 hours. Chronic urticaria lasts more than 6 consecutive weeks and negatively influences the patient's quality of life. Its etiology is not well determined, drugs, foods, malignancies, and autoimmune disease are incriminated, but in many patients, no etiological factors are detected. A study on urticaria patients found HP antigens in 69% of the study group [22]. Other studies did not find any difference between the occurrence rate of HP in chronic urticaria but found a statistically significant clinical improvement in the urticaria symptoms in those patients treated for HP. A slow urticaria symptoms rebound phenomenon was observed after 6 weeks post HP eradication therapy, possibly due to reinfection [23].

Rosacea is an inflammatory skin disease affecting the central part of the face. It presents as a mixture of papules, pustules, erythema, and telangiectasias. Its etiology is unknown. Epidemiological studies found an association between HP infection and the development of rosacea. Two mechanisms through which HP produces the rosacea skin lesions were identified: the increase of nitrous oxide at the skin level (responsible for inflammation, vasodilatation, and immune stimulation) and specific cytotoxic reaction [24]. Associating HP eradication treatment with routine treatment in these patients showed a better effect than routine therapy alone [25].

Psoriasis is a chronic skin disease presenting as erythema, papules, and scales. The lesions appear usually on the elbows and knees but can involve other skin areas too. It greatly influences the patient's quality of life and up to date, no cure has been found.

Symptomatic treatment can help in controlling the clinical manifestations. HP infections are statistically associated with psoriasis while psoriasis patients with HP infection seem to have a higher Psoriasis Severity Score Index [26] showing a contribution of HP in the development of psoriasis, while no data is available concerning the possibility of psoriasis making patients more prone to HP infections. A recent nationwide population-based cohort study on 41,500 patients with HP infection showed no association between HP and psoriasis, therefore further studies are needed to reach a conclusion [27].

In psoriasis patients with HP infection, eradicating the infection ameliorates psoriasis severity and the patients treated for both psoriasis and HP present rapid improvement compared to patients only treated for psoriasis [28, 29].

HP does not seem to be a causative factor in dermatological diseases, but HP eradication improves symptoms and positively impacts treatment results in these diseases, raising the theory of HP being a trigger for several chronic skin diseases.

4. Ophthalmic diseases

Central serous chorioretinopathy is usually unilateral and it is characterized by the presence of liquid accumulation under the macula. The visual acuity is reduced and the vision is blurred and distorted. In most cases, it is self-limited, but chronic, non-resolving, and recurrent forms are possible in 15% of patients [30]. The prevalence of HP infection in these patients was determined to be 2.5-fold higher compared to the control groups [31].

Treating the HP infection (if present) in patients with central serous chorioretinopathy proved to decrease both the duration of the disease and the rate of recurrence while improving distant prognosis [32].

Open-angle glaucoma is a disease of the optic nerve head associated with increased intraocular pressure. It is one of the most frequent causes of blindness worldwide. In 2000 a study confirmed the association of HP gastric infection with glaucoma in 88% of glaucoma patients. Later studies found the same association [33]. A meta-analysis including 2664 participants showed a positive association between HP and open-angle glaucoma [34].

Giving treatment for HP infection has not yet been proven to improve or cure open-angle glaucoma, but studies seem promising. Reduction in intraocular pressure was found after 2 months in glaucoma patients who received HP eradication therapy [35].

Blepharitis is a chronic inflammation of the eyelid margin that causes ocular irritation. It is one of the most common ophthalmic diseases [36]. Its connection with HP infection is not clearly determined. A study conducted on 186 patients with blepharitis showed an increased incidence of HP infection compared to the control group; the symptoms were more severe in HP-positive patients, and a clinical improvement in 50% of the patients treated for HP was observed. As both conditions are highly prevalent in the population, their relationship needs large studies in order to be exactly determined [37].

5. Hematological diseases

The association of HP infection with *iron deficiency anemia* is well documented. The guidelines for the treatment of HP state the necessity of eradicating HP infection in patients with iron deficiency anemia [38]. Hepcidin (a protein produced in the liver) has been studied as the key mechanism. This protein is responsible for the iron balance in the organism, regulating its intestinal absorption and its release from the macrophages [39, 40]. HP infection upregulates the levels of hepcidin, in this case, treatment with iron is less efficient [41]. Also, the higher gastric acidity in HP infection decreases dietary iron absorption. HP gastric lesions bleeding can also be a cause of anemia [42, 43].

Primary immune thrombocytopenia (autoimmune thrombocytopenic purpura) is an autoimmune disease characterized by an isolated low blood platelet count whose cause cannot be determined. Many studies have reported the association of this type of thrombocytopenia with HP infection. The pathogenic mechanism is complex. Eradication of HP in these patients proved to increase platelet count by 26–100% [43–46].

Chronic vitamin B12 deficiency leading to *pernicious anemia*, peripheral neuropathy, and spinal cord lesions can be associated with HP infection [47]. The absorption of B12 at the gastric level is reduced in HP-related gastritis of the corpus. HP eradication treatment increases serum levels of B12 and decreases serum homocysteine (a component of the metabolic pathway of B12) [43].

Chronic idiopathic neutropenia's association with HP infection was confirmed in several studies. These findings suggest that testing for HP in these patients and eradicating the infection can be beneficial [48, 49].

6. Cardio-vascular diseases

Coronary atherosclerosis and *myocardial infarction* are the most frequent causes of mortality in many countries. There are well-known risk factors: hypertension, diabetes, obesity, dyslipidemia, smoking, and family history, but they are not present in all patients [50, 51]. Other causes need to be investigated in order to improve treatment and prevention.

Extensive metanalysis on 20,900 participants showed a correlation between HP and coronary atherosclerosis, even when various HP-detecting methods were used (anti-HP IgG, positive anti-CagA, positive HP stool antigen, positive HP histological staining) [52]. The correlation is even stronger in patients with myocardial infarction [53].

The mechanism by which HP can cause coronary heart disease is complex. HP in the atherosclerotic plaque stimulates inflammatory cells, which produce cytokines. They determine endothelial and vascular dysfunction. HP also increases the production of interleukin 1 and 6, C-reactive protein, and TNF-α. These substances cause instability in the atherosclerotic plaque. HP secretes vacuolating cytotoxin A, which reduces nitric oxide concentration and further damages the endothelial function. HP infection also increases platelet aggregation [54–58].

Eradication treatment in these patients seems to be beneficial. Early HP treatment introduction, especially in younger patients (<65 years) patients improved survival and decreased the appearance of coronary heart disease. The benefit was modest when HP treatment was given to older patients [59].

Chronic *arterial hypertension* is one of the most common diseases worldwide. It is considered a global public health problem, leading to a multitude of serious complications [60]. A positive association with HP has been found, although no correlation was evident between the grades of hypertension and HP infection status [61–63].

HP eradication treatment in infected hypertensive patients proved to reduce the blood pressure values, even to normal values in some cases [64, 65].

7. Metabolic diseases

Diabetes is the most frequent disease worldwide. Studies have found that HP infection increases an individual's risk of having type 1 or type 2 diabetes. There seems to be a correlation between HP infection and the levels of glycated hemoglobin in diabetic patients [66]. HP infection in patients with type 1 diabetes was associated with poorer glycemic control compared to patients without HP. Eradication of HP in these patients did not improve glycemic values in a short time follow-up [67].

Studies have shown an improvement in glucose homeostasis in patients with type 2 diabetes after HP eradication [68, 69].

Metabolic syndrome has five components: central obesity, high blood glucose (insulin resistance), high triglycerides, low HDL, and high blood pressure. In order to establish the diagnosis of metabolic syndrome, at least three of the components have to be present. The disorders are evaluated by measuring the following: fasting glucose levels, triglycerides levels, HDL levels, cholesterol levels, blood pressure, and waist circumference. The presence of this syndrome elevates the risk of an individual developing atherosclerotic cardiovascular disease, diabetes mellitus, and neurological and vascular complications [70, 71].

HP infection determines chronic inflammation and immune response. Inflammatory cytokines and adipokines are present. HP induces low leptin and high TNF-α in infected patients. This leads to insulin resistance, which is an important component of the metabolic syndrome [72–74].

Several studies have addressed this correlation. They showed that people with obesity had a 46% increase in the chance of being infected with HP compared to normal weight controls. The chance of diabetic patients to develop an HP infection is 27% higher than non-diabetic persons [75, 76]. Several studies have shown a correlation between HP infection and metabolic syndrome [77–80]. Nevertheless, there are a small number of studies that found no statistical association between them [81, 82].

The question of the benefit of HP eradication treatment on metabolic syndrome components has been investigated. A study showed beneficial change after treatment, with a reduction in total cholesterol, and LDL, an increase of HDL, and a reduction in waist circumference. No influence was seen on body weight, blood pressure, and triglyceride values [83].

In a South Korean study, 2267 subjects were followed for 5 years after HP eradication. The follow-up focused on metabolic parameters. The results showed that HP treatment significantly increased HDL in female patients, especially at the 1st year follow-up. Body mass index increased in males over time. No statistically significant influence was found for other factors [84]. A study conducted in Taiwan showed significant improvement in metabolic parameters after eradication treatment [85].

8. COVID-19

Although not a causative factor for COVID-19, recent studies have targeted a possible interaction between SARS-CoV-2 infection and concomitant HP presence in patients. The association of these two pathogens seems to make patients more prone to severe forms with digestive manifestations of COVID-19 [86].

In patients with both infections, there was no statistically significant difference in the severity of common symptoms (fever, dry cough, dyspnea, loss of taste, loss of smell headache, nausea, vomiting) compared to COVID-19 patients without HP infection [86].

Patients with HP use a lot of anti-acid and acid-reducing medicine (proton pump inhibitors), which leads to a higher gastric pH. Gastric acidity is considered to offer digestive protection for COVID-19, so in these patients stopping the anti-acid and related medicine might be considered during the acute phase of COVID-19 [87].

The vascular endothelium is an important factor in vascular homeostasis, it regulates fibrinolysis, blood viscosity, monocyte/leucocyte adhesion, and angiogenesis. Endothelial vascular cells regulate inflammatory response at inflammation sites. Markers of vascular endothelial dysfunction (V-CAM, ICAM, TNF-α, IL-8, IL-1β) were present in severe forms of COVID-19 [88, 89]. Inflammatory activation is also caused by HP infection, so a strong inflammatory response can be seen in patients with both pathogens, leading to severe forms of COVID-19 [90].

In future studies, as more SARS-COV2 data will be available, more information concerning the results and consequences of the coexistence of these two infections will be discovered, leading to a better treatment choice.

9. Conclusions

Helicobacter pylori's implication in human disease goes beyond gastric localization. Studies have shown its detrimental effect on various types of diseases, from neurological and hematological, to skin and metabolism.

The mechanisms through which HP contributes to the pathogenesis or influences the severity of extra gastric diseases are complex and partially understood, but they seem to have a common pathway-systemic inflammation. HP infection determines the release of proinflammatory factors (e.g., IL-1, IL-6, TNF, C-reactive protein) which lead to chronic inflammation. Chronic inflammation contributes to several chronic diseases affecting different organs and systems, such as dermatological, cardio-vascular hematological, metabolic, ophthalmic, and COVID-19. This mechanism seems to be similar in most chronic neurological diseases, except for multiple sclerosis, where the change of immune profile induced by HP infection, leading to an increase of Treg may have, according to some studies, a favorable effect on disease progression by reducing demyelination. Also, HP gastric infection can influence the response to treatment in certain diseases by decreasing drug absorption.

Future studies will give more information and will help in providing better treatment strategies for a lot of different diseases. Large-scale studies will provide even better information in this domain and molecular studies will give more information on etiopathogenic mechanisms.

Doctors of all specialties should take into consideration the possible presence of HP and consider its implications. They should evaluate the potential beneficial effect of eradication treatment upon the evolution of the disease they are treating or the health risk reduction it might provide.

Conflict of interest

The authors declare no conflict of interest.

Author details

Mihaela-Flavia Avram[1,2]*, Daniela Cornelia Lazăr[3] and Sorin Olariu[1,2]

1 Department of Surgery X, 1st Surgery Discipline, "Victor Babeş" University of Medicine and Pharmacy Timişoara, Romania

2 Abdominal Surgery and Phlebology Research Center, "Victor Babes" University of Medicine and Pharmacy Timisoara, Timisoara, Romania

3 Department V of Internal Medicine I, Discipline of Internal Medicine IV, "Victor Babeş" University of Medicine and Pharmacy Timişoara, Romania

*Address all correspondence to: avram.mihaela@umft.ro

References

[1] Mendall MA, Goggin PM, Molineaux N, et al. Relation of helicobacter pylori infection and coronary heart disease. British Heart Journal. 1994;**71**(5):437-439. DOI: 10.1136/hrt.71.5.437

[2] Daugule I, Zavoronkova J, Santare D. *Helicobacter pylori* and allergy: Update of research. WJM. 2015;**5**:203. DOI: 10.5662/wjm.v5.i4.203

[3] Park A-M, Omura S, Fujita M, Sato F, Tsunoda I. *Helicobacter pylori* and gut microbiota in multiple sclerosis versus Alzheimer's disease: 10 pitfalls of microbiome studies. Clinical & Experimental Neuroimmunology. 2017;**8**:215-232. DOI: 10.1111/cen3.12401

[4] Jaruvongvanich V, Sanguankeo A, Jaruvongvanich S, Upala S. Association between *Helicobacter pylori* infection and multiple sclerosis: A systematic review and meta-analysis. Multiple Sclerosis and Related Disorders. 2016;7:92-97. DOI: 10.1016/j.msard.2016.03.013

[5] Xu Y, Wang Q, Liu Y, Cui R, Zhao Y. Is *Helicobacter pylori* infection a critical risk factor for vascular dementia? The International Journal of Neuroscience. 2016;**126**:899-903. DOI: 10.3109/00207454.2015.1081387

[6] Jackson L, Britton J, Lewis SA, McKeever TM, Atherton J, Fullerton D, et al. A population-based epidemiologic study of *Helicobacter pylori* infection and its association with systemic inflammation. Helicobacter. 2009;**14**:460-465. DOI: 10.1111/j.1523-5378.2009.00711.x

[7] Park AM, Tsunoda I. *Helicobacter pylori* infection in the stomach induces neuroinflammation: The potential roles of bacterial outer membrane vesicles in an animal model of Alzheimer's disease. Inflammation and Regeneration. 2022;**42**(1):39. DOI: 10.1186/s41232-022-00224-8

[8] Dobbs RJ, Dobbs SM, Weller C, Charlett A, Bjarnason IT, Curry A, et al. *Helicobacter* hypothesis for idiopathic parkinsonism: Before and beyond. Helicobacter. 2008;**13**:309-322. DOI: 10.1111/j.1523-5378.2008.00622.x

[9] Katsinelos T, Doulberis M, Polyzos SA, Papaefthymiou A, Katsinelos P, Kountouras J. Molecular links between Alzheimer's disease and gastrointestinal microbiota: Emphasis on helicobacter pylori infection involvement. Current Molecular Medicine. 2019;**20**(1):3-12. DOI: 10.2174/1566524019666190917125917

[10] Roubaud-Baudron C, Krolak-Salmon P, Quadrio I, Mégraud F, Salles N. Impact of chronic *Helicobacter pylori* infection on Alzheimer's disease: Preliminary results. Neurobiology of Aging. 2012;**33**(5):1009.e11-1009.e1.009E19. DOI: 10.1016/j.neurobiolaging.2011.10.021

[11] BeydounMA, BeydounHA, ShroffMR, Kitner-Triolo MH, Zonderman AB. *Helicobacter pylori* seropositivity and cognitive performance among US adults: Evidence from a large national survey. Psychosomatic Medicine. 2013;**75**(5):486-496. DOI: 10.1097/PSY.0b013e31829108c3

[12] Kountouras J, Boziki M, Gavalas E, et al. Five-year survival after *Helicobacter pylori* eradication in Alzheimer disease patients. Cognitive and Behavioral Neurology. 2010;**23**(3):199-204. DOI: 10.1097/WNN.0b013e3181df3034

[13] Ritz K, Denswil NP, Stam OC, van Lieshout JJ, Daemen MJ. Cause and mechanisms of intracranial atherosclerosis. Circulation. 2014;**130**(16):1407-1414. DOI: 10.1161/CIRCULATIONAHA.114.011147

[14] Doheim MF, Altaweel AA, Elgendy MG, et al. Association between *Helicobacter pylori* infection and stroke: A meta-analysis of 273,135 patients. Journal of Neurology. 2021;**268**(9):3238-3248. DOI: 10.1007/s00415-020-09933-x

[15] Guo Y, Xu C, Zhang L, Chen Z, Xia X. *Helicobacter pylori* infection acts as an independent risk factor for intracranial atherosclerosis in women less than 60 years old. Frontiers in Cardiovascular Medicine. 2022;**8**:819315. DOI: 10.3389/fcvm.2021.819315 [Accessed: Jan 11, 2022]

[16] Kira JI, Isobe N. *Helicobacter pylori* infection and demyelinating disease of the central nervous system. Journal of Neuroimmunology. 2019;**329**:14-19. DOI: 10.1016/j.jneuroim.2018.06.017

[17] Yao G, Wang P, Luo XD, Yu TM, Harris RA, Zhang XM. Meta-analysis of association between *Helicobacter pylori* infection and multiple sclerosis. Neuroscience Letters. 2016;**620**:1-7. DOI: 10.1016/j.neulet.2016.03.037

[18] Cook KW, Crooks J, Hussain K, et al. *Helicobacter pylori* infection reduces disease severity in an experimental model of multiple sclerosis. Frontiers in Microbiology. 2015;**6**:52. DOI: 10.3389/fmicb.2015.00052 [Accessed: Feb 13, 2015]

[19] Baj J, Forma A, Flieger W, et al. *Helicobacter pylori* infection and extragastric diseases—A focus on the central nervous system. Cells. 2021;**10**(9):2191. [Accessed: Aug 25, 2021]. DOI: 10.3390/cells10092191

[20] Mridula KR, Borgohain R, Chandrasekhar Reddy V, Bandaru VC, Suryaprabha T. Association of Helicobacter pylori with Parkinson's disease. Journal of Clinical Neurology. 2017;**13**(2):181-186. DOI: 10.3988/jcn.2017.13.2.181

[21] Lolekha P, Sriphanom T, Vilaichone RK. *Helicobacter pylori* eradication improves motor fluctuations in advanced Parkinson's disease patients: A prospective cohort study (HP-PD trial). PLoS One. 2021;**16**(5):e0251042. DOI: 10.1371/journal.pone.0251042 [Accessed: May 4, 2021]

[22] Erdem Y, Altunay I, Ozkur E, Sivaz O. The etiological evaluation of patients with chronic urticaria. Sisli Etfal Hastanesi Tip Bülteni. 2020;**54**(4):424-427. DOI: 10.14744/SEMB.2018.98216 [Accessed: Dec 11, 2020]

[23] Pawłowicz R, Wytrychowski K, Panaszek B. Eradication of *Helicobacter pylori*, as add-on therapy, has a significant, but temporary influence on recovery in chronic idiopathic urticaria: A placebo-controlled, double blind trial in the Polish population. Postępy Dermatologii i Alergologii. 2018;**35**(2):151-155. DOI: 10.5114/ada.2018.75236

[24] Bhattarai S, Agrawal S, Rijal A, Majhi S, Pradhan B, Dhakal S. The study of prevalence of helicobacter pylori in patients with acne rosacea. Kathmandu University Medical Journal. 2014;**10**(4):49-52. DOI: 10.3126/kumj.v10i4.10995

[25] Yang X. Relationship between *Helicobacter pylori* and Rosacea: Review and discussion. BMC Infectious Diseases. 2018;**18**(1):318. DOI: 10.1186/s12879-018-3232-4 [Accessed: Jul 11, 2018]

[26] Yu M, Zhang R, Ni P, Chen S, Duan G. *Helicobacter pylori* infection

and psoriasis: A systematic review and meta-analysis. Medicina (Kaunas). 2019;**55**(10):645. DOI: 10.3390/medicina55100645 [Accessed: Sep 26, 2019]

[27] Wu MC, Ma KS, Chen HH, Huang JY, Wei JC. Relationship between *Helicobacter pylori* infection and psoriasis: A nationwide population-based longitudinal cohort study. Medicine (Baltimore). 2020;**99**(24):e20632. DOI: 10.1097/MD.0000000000020632

[28] Onsun N, Arda Ulusal H, Su O, Beycan I, Biyik Ozkaya D, Senocak M. Impact of *Helicobacter pylori* infection on severity of psoriasis and response to treatment. European Journal of Dermatology. 2012;**22**(1):117-120. DOI: 10.1684/ejd.2011.1579

[29] Ahmed AS, Al-Najjar AH, Alshalahi H, Altowayan WM, Elgharabawy RM. Clinical significance of *Helicobacter pylori* infection on psoriasis severity. Journal of Interferon & Cytokine Research. 2021;**41**(2):44-51. DOI: 10.1089/jir.2020.0144

[30] Sartini F, Figus M, Nardi M, Casini G, Posarelli C. Non-resolving, recurrent and chronic central serous chorioretinopathy: Available treatment options. Eye (London, England). 2019;**33**(7):1035-1043. DOI: 10.1038/s41433-019-0381-7

[31] Bagheri M, Rashe Z, Ahoor MH, Somi MH. Prevalence of *Helicobacter pylori* infection in patients with central serous chorioretinopathy: A review. Medical Hypothesis, Discovery & Innovation in Ophthalmology. 2017;**6**(4):118-124

[32] Zavoloka O, Bezditko P, Lahorzhevska I, Zubkova D, Ilyina Y. Clinical efficiency of *Helicobacter pylori* eradication in the treatment of patients with acute central serous chorioretinopathy. Graefe's Archive for Clinical and Experimental Ophthalmology. 2016;**254**(9):1737-1742. DOI: 10.1007/s00417-016-3315-0

[33] Kountouras J, Mylopoulos N, Boura P, et al. Relationship between *Helicobacter pylori* infection and glaucoma. Ophthalmology. 2001;**108**(3):599-604. DOI: 10.1016/s0161-6420(00)00598-4

[34] Doulberis M, Papaefthymiou A, Polyzos SA, et al. Association between active *Helicobacter pylori* infection and glaucoma: A systematic review and meta-analysis. Microorganisms. 2020;**8**(6):894. DOI: 10.3390/microorganisms8060894. [Accessed: Jun 13, 2020]

[35] Ala S, Maleki I, Sanjari Araghi A, Sahebnasagh A, Shahraki A. *Helicobacter pylori* eradication in the management of glaucoma. Caspian Journal of Internal Medicine. 2020;**11**(2):143-149. DOI: 10.22088/cjim.11.2.143

[36] Amescua G, Akpek EK, Farid M, et al. Blepharitis preferred practice pattern®. Ophthalmology. 2019;**126**(1):P56-P93. DOI: 10.1016/j.ophtha.2018.10.019

[37] Saccà SC, Pascotto A, Venturino GM, et al. Prevalence and treatment of *Helicobacter pylori* in patients with blepharitis. Investigative Ophthalmology & Visual Science. 2006;**47**(2):501-508. DOI: 10.1167/iovs.05-0323

[38] Malfertheiner P, Megraud F, O'Morain CA, et al. Management of *Helicobacter pylori* infection-the Maastricht V/Florence consensus report. Gut. 2017;**66**(1):6-30. DOI: 10.1136/gutjnl-2016-312288

[39] Ozkasap S, Yarali N, Isik P, Bay A, Kara A, Tunc B. The role of prohepcidin in anemia due to *Helicobacter pylori*

infection. Pediatric Hematology and Oncology. 2013;**30**(5):425-431. DOI: 10.3109/08880018.2013.783144

[40] Senkovich O, Ceaser S, McGee DJ, Testerman TL. Unique host iron utilization mechanisms of *Helicobacter pylori* revealed with iron-deficient chemically defined media. Infection and Immunity. 2010;**78**(5):1841-1849. DOI: 10.1128/IAI.01258-09

[41] Kroot JJ, Tjalsma H, Fleming RE, Swinkels DW. Hepcidin in human iron disorders: Diagnostic implications. Clinical Chemistry. 2011;**57**(12):1650-1669. DOI: 10.1373/clinchem.2009.140053

[42] De Leest HT, Steen KS, Bloemena E, et al. *Helicobacter pylori* eradication in patients on long-term treatment with NSAIDs reduces the severity of gastritis: A randomized controlled trial. Journal of Clinical Gastroenterology. 2009;**43**(2):140-146. DOI: 10.1097/MCG.0b013e3181595b40

[43] Campuzano-Maya G. Hematologic manifestations of *Helicobacter pylori* infection. World Journal of Gastroenterology. 2014;**20**(36):12818-12838. DOI: 10.3748/wjg.v20.i36.12818

[44] Stasi R, Rossi Z, Stipa E, Amadori S, Newland AC, Provan D. *Helicobacter pylori* eradication in the management of patients with idiopathic thrombocytopenic purpura. The American Journal of Medicine. 2005;**118**(4):414-419. DOI: 10.1016/j.amjmed.2004.09.014

[45] Suvajdzić N, Stanković B, Artiko V, et al. *Helicobacter pylori* eradication can induce platelet recovery in chronic idiopathic thrombocytopenic purpura. Platelets. 2006;**17**(4):227-230. DOI: 10.1080/09537100500462487

[46] Jackson SC, Beck P, Buret AG, et al. Long term platelet responses to *Helicobacter pylori* eradication in Canadian patients with immune thrombocytopenic purpura. International Journal of Hematology. 2008;**88**(2):212-218. DOI: 10.1007/s12185-008-0138-8

[47] Lahner E, Persechino S, Annibale B. Micronutrients (other than iron) and *Helicobacter pylori* infection: A systematic review. Helicobacter. 2012;**17**(1):1-15. DOI: 10.1111/j.1523-5378.2011.00892.x

[48] Wang L, Zou X, Liu YF, Sheng GY. Association between *Helicobacter pylori* infection and chronic idiopathic neutropenia. Journal of Huazhong University of Science and Technology. Medical Sciences. 2013;**33**(3):353-356. DOI: 10.1007/s11596-013-1123-x

[49] Papadaki HA, Pontikoglou C, Stavroulaki E, et al. High prevalence of *Helicobacter pylori* infection and monoclonal gammopathy of undetermined significance in patients with chronic idiopathic neutropenia. Annals of Hematology. 2005;**84**(5):317-320. DOI: 10.1007/s00277-004-0996-y

[50] Virani SS, Alonso A, Benjamin EJ, Bittencourt MS, Callaway CW, Carson AP, et al. Heart disease and stroke statistics-2020 update: A report from the American heart association. Circulation. 2020;**141**:e139-e596. DOI: 10.1161/CIR.0000000000000007

[51] Helfand M, Buckley DI, Freeman M, Fu R, Rogers K, Fleming C, et al. Emerging risk factors for coronary heart disease: A summary of systematic reviews conducted for the U.S. preventive services task force. Annals of Internal Medicine. 2009;**151**:496-507. DOI: 10.7326/0003-4819-151-7-200910060-00010

[52] Tong L, Wang BB, Li FH, Lv SP, Pan FF, Dong XJ. An updated meta-analysis of the relationship between

Helicobacter pylori infection and the risk of coronary heart disease. Frontiers in Cardiovascular Medicine. 2022;**9**:794445. DOI: 10.3389/fcvm.2022.794445 [Accessed: Apr 29, 2022]

[53] Wang B, Yu M, Zhang R, Chen S, Xi Y, Duan G. A meta-analysis of the association between *Helicobacter pylori* infection and risk of atherosclerotic cardiovascular disease. Helicobacter. 2020;**25**:e12761. DOI: 10.1111/hel.12761

[54] Kinjo K, Sato H, Sato H, Shiotani I, Kurotobi T, Ohnishi Y, et al. Prevalence of *Helicobacter pylori* infection and its link to coronary risk factors in Japanese patients with acute myocardial infarction. Circulation Journal. 2002;**66**:805-810. DOI: 10.1253/circj.66.805

[55] Figura N, Palazzuoli A, Vaira D, Campagna M, Moretti E, Iacoponi F, et al. Cross-sectional study: CagA-positive *Helicobacter pylori* infection, acute coronary artery disease and systemic levels of B-type natriuretic peptide. Journal of Clinical Pathology. 2014;**67**:251-257. DOI: 10.1136/jclinpath-2013-201743

[56] Xia XJ, Zhang LF, Chi JS, Li H, Liu XM, Hu TZ, et al. *Helicobacter pylori* infection impairs endothelial function through an exosome-mediated mechanism. Journal of the American Heart Association. 2020;**9**:e014120. DOI: 10.1161/JAHA.119.014120

[57] Tobin NP, Henehan GT, Murphy RP, Atherton JC, Guinan AF, Kerrigan SW, et al. *Helicobacter pylori*-induced inhibition of vascular endothelial cell functions: A role for VacA-dependent nitric oxide reduction. American Journal of Physiology. Heart and Circulatory Physiology. 2008;**295**:H1403-H1413. DOI: 10.1152/ajpheart.00240.2008

[58] Yeh JJ, Tsai S, Wu DC, Wu JY, Liu TC, Chen A. P-selectin-dependent platelet aggregation and apoptosis may explain the decrease in platelet count during *Helicobacter pylori* infection. Blood. 2010;**115**:4247-4253. DOI: 10.1182/blood-2009-09-241166

[59] Wang JW, Tseng KL, Hsu CN, et al. Association between *Helicobacter pylori* eradication and the risk of coronary heart diseases. PLoS One. 2018;**13**(1):e0190219. DOI: 10.1371/journal.pone.0190219 [Accessed: Jan 2, 2018]

[60] Subasinghe AK, Arabshahi S, Busingye D, et al. Association between salt and hypertension in rural and urban populations of low to middle income countries: A systematic review and meta-analysis of population based studies. Asia Pacific Journal of Clinical Nutrition. 2016;**25**(2):402-413. DOI: 10.6133/apjcn.2016.25.2.25

[61] Wan Z, Hu L, Hu M, Lei X, Huang Y, Lv Y. *Helicobacter pylori* infection and prevalence of high blood pressure among Chinese adults. Journal of Human Hypertension. 2018;**32**(2):158-164. DOI: 10.1038/s41371-017-0028-8

[62] Lu C, Jia H, Xu A, et al. *Helicobacter pylori* infection and pepsinogen levels have clinical significance in hypertension patients. International Journal of Clinical and Experimental Medicine. 2014;**7**(12):5675-5680 [Accessed: Dec 15, 2014]

[63] Huang M, Zhu L, Jin Y, Fang Z, Chen Y, Yao Y. Association between *Helicobacter pylori* infection and systemic arterial hypertension: A meta-analysis. Associação entre Infecção por Heicobacter Pylori e Hipertensão Arterial Sistêmica: Metanálise: Arquivos Brasileiros de Cardiologia. 2021;**117**(4):626-636. DOI: 10.36660/abc.20200186

[64] Nasrat SA, Nasrat AM. An alternative approach for the rising challenge of hypertensive illness via *Helicobacter pylori* eradication. Cardiology Research. 2015;**6**(1):221-225. DOI: 10.14740/cr382e

[65] Migneco A, Ojetti V, Specchia L, et al. Eradication of *Helicobacter pylori* infection improves blood pressure values in patients affected by hypertension. Helicobacter. 2003;**8**(6):585-589. DOI: 10.1111/j.1523-5378.2003.00180.x

[66] Chen J, Xing Y, Zhao L, Ma H. The association between *Helicobacter pylori* infection and glycated hemoglobin a in diabetes: A meta-analysis. Journal Diabetes Research. 2019;**2019**:3705264. DOI: 10.1155/2019/3705264 [Accessed: Sep 9, 2019]

[67] Dai YN, Yu WL, Zhu HT, Ding JX, Yu CH, Li YM. Is *Helicobacter pylori* infection associated with glycemic control in diabetics? World Journal of Gastroenterology. 2015;**21**(17):5407-5416. DOI: 10.3748/wjg.v21.i17.5407

[68] Bonfigli AR, Boemi M, Festa R, et al. Randomized, double-blind, placebo-controlled trial to evaluate the effect of *Helicobacter pylori* eradication on glucose homeostasis in type 2 diabetic patients. Nutrition, Metabolism, and Cardiovascular Diseases. 2016;**26**(10):893-898. DOI: 10.1016/j.numecd.2016.06.012

[69] Song X, Cai C, Jin Q, Chen X, Yu C. The efficacy of *Helicobacter pylori* eradication in diabetics and its effect on glycemic control: A systematic review and meta-analysis. Helicobacter. 2021;**26**(2):e12781. DOI: 10.1111/hel.12781

[70] Swarup S, Goyal A, Grigorova Y, Zeltser R. Metabolic syndrome. In: StatPearls. Treasure Island (FL): StatPearls Publishing; 2022

[71] Fahed G, Aoun L, Bou Zerdan M, et al. Metabolic syndrome: Updates on pathophysiology and management in 2021. International Journal of Molecular Sciences. 2022;**23**(2):786. DOI: 10.3390/ijms23020786

[72] Shoelson SE, Herrero L, Naaz A. Obesity, inflammation, and insulin resistance. Gastroenterology. 2007;**132**(6):2169-2180. DOI: 10.1053/j.gastro.2007.03.059

[73] Kusters JG, van Vliet AH, Kuipers EJ. Pathogenesis of *Helicobacter pylori* infection. Clinical Microbiology Reviews. 2006;**19**(3):449-490. DOI: 10.1128/CMR.00054-05

[74] Thalmaier U, Lehn N, Pfeffer K, Stolte M, Vieth M, Schneider-Brachert W. Role of tumor necrosis factor alpha in *Helicobacter pylori* gastritis in tumor necrosis factor receptor 1-deficient mice. Infection and Immunity. 2002;**70**(6):3149-3155. DOI: 10.1128/IAI.70.6.3149-3155.2002

[75] Baradaran A, Dehghanbanadaki H, Naderpour S, et al. The association between *Helicobacter pylori* and obesity: A systematic review and meta-analysis of case–control studies. Clinical Diabetes and Endocrinology. 2021;7:15. DOI: 10.1186/s40842-021-00131-w

[76] Mansori K, Moradi Y, Naderpour S, et al. *Helicobacter pylori* infection as a risk factor for diabetes: A meta-analysis of case-control studies. BMC Gastroenterology. 2020;**20**:77. DOI: 10.1186/s12876-020-01223-0

[77] Jeon CY, Haan MN, Cheng C, et al. *Helicobacter pylori* infection is associated with an increased rate of diabetes. Diabetes Care. 2012;**35**(3):520-525. DOI: 10.2337/dc11-1043

[78] Kayar Y, Pamukçu Ö, Eroğlu H, Kalkan Erol K, Ilhan A, Kocaman O.

Relationship between *Helicobacter pylori* infections in diabetic patients and inflammations, metabolic syndrome, and complications. International Journal of Chronic Diseases. 2015;**2015**:290128. DOI: 10.1155/2015/290128

[79] Sayılar EI, Çelik B, Dumlu Ş. Relationship between *Helicobacter pylori* infection and metabolic syndrome. The Turkish Journal of Gastroenterology. 2015;**26**(6):468-473

[80] Azami M, Baradaran HR, Dehghanbanadaki H, et al. Association of *Helicobacter pylori* infection with the risk of metabolic syndrome and insulin resistance: An updated systematic review and meta-analysis. Diabetology & Metabolic Syndrome. 2021;**13**(1):145. DOI: 10.1186/s13098-021-00765-x [Accessed: Dec 18, 2021]

[81] Zhou F, Zhong X, Chen J, et al. *Helicobacter pylori* infection associated with type 2 diabetic nephropathy in patients with dyspeptic symptoms. Diabetes Research and Clinical Practice. 2015;**110**(3):328-334. DOI: 10.1016/j.diabres.2015.09.008

[82] Han X, Li Y, Wang J, et al. *Helicobacter pylori* infection is associated with type 2 diabetes among a middle- and old-age Chinese population. Diabetes/Metabolism Research and Reviews. 2016;**32**(1):95-101. DOI: 10.1002/dmrr.2677

[83] Mokhtare M, Mirfakhraee H, Arshad M, et al. The effects of *Helicobacter pylori* eradication on modification of metabolic syndrome parameters in patients with functional dyspepsia. Diabetes and Metabolic Syndrome: Clinical Research and Reviews. 2017;**11**(Suppl. 2):S1031-S1035. DOI: 10.1016/j.dsx.2017.07.035

[84] Park J, Kim N, Kim WS, et al. Long-term effects of the eradication of *Helicobacter pylori* on metabolic parameters, depending on sex, in South Korea. Gut Liver. 2022. DOI: 10.5009/gnl210588. Published online ahead of print [Accessed: Jun 30, 2022]

[85] Liou JM, Chen CC, Chang CM, et al. Long-term changes of gut microbiota, antibiotic resistance, and metabolic parameters after helicobacter pylori eradication: A multicentre, open-label, randomised trial. The Lancet Infectious Diseases. 2019;**19**(10):1109-1120. DOI: 10.1016/S1473-3099(19)30272-5

[86] Balamtekin N, Artuk C, Arslan M, Gülşen M. The effect of *Helicobacter pylori* on the presentation and clinical course of coronavirus disease 2019 infection. Journal of Pediatric Gastroenterology and Nutrition. 2021;**72**(4):511-513. DOI: 10.1097/MPG.0000000000003005

[87] Price E. Could the severity of COVID-19 be increased by low gastric acidity? Critical Care. 2020;**24**(1):456. DOI: 10.1186/s13054-020-03182-0 [Accessed: Jul 22, 2020]

[88] Hang W, Chen C, Zhang XA, Wang DW. Endothelial dysfunction in COVID-19 calls for immediate attention: The emerging roles of the endothelium in inflammation caused by SARS-CoV-2. Frontiers in Medicine. 2021;**15**(4):638-643. DOI: 10.1007/s11684-021-0831-z

[89] Libby P, Lüscher T. COVID-19 is, in the end, an endothelial disease. European Heart Journal. 2020;**41**(32):3038-3044. DOI: 10.1093/eurheartj/ehaa623

[90] He J, Liu Y, Ouyang Q, et al. *Helicobacter pylori* and unignorable extragastric diseases: Mechanism and implications. Frontiers in Microbiology. 2022;**13**:972777. DOI: 10.3389/fmicb.2022.972777. [Accessed: Aug 4, 2022]

Chapter 5

Changes in Vitamin B_{12}, Iron, Thyroid Hormones, Thyroid Autoantibodies and Hematological Indices Levels in Patients Suffering from *Helicobacter pylori* Infection

Saleh Nazmy Mwafy, Wesam Mohammad Afana and Asma'a Ali Hejaze

Abstract

Helicobacter pylori infection has been recognized as a public health problem worldwide with raising prevalence in developing than the developed countries. More than 50% of the world's population infected, and 80% of infected have no symptoms. Megaloblastic anemia can occur due to impaired DNA synthesis resulting from deficiencies of vitamin B_{12} and folate. The development of autoantibodies to thyroid peroxidase (anti-TPO), thyroglobulin (anti-Tg), and thyroid-stimulating hormone receptor (TSH-R) is the main characteristic of autoimmune thyroid disease. *H. pylori* may decrease absorption of oral thyroxine by decreasing gastric acid secretion in the stomach. *H. pylori* has important role of in the development of autoimmune thyroid diseases, vitamin B_{12} deficiency and malfunctions of human. The primary goal of this chapter is to observe association between *H. pylori* infection in the gastric mucosa and of autoimmune thyroid diseases vitamin B_{12} deficiency because eradication of *H. pylori* can prevent the development of complications.

Keywords: vitamin B_{12}, iron, thyroid hormones, thyroid autoantibodies, *Helicobacter pylori*

1. Introduction

Helicobacter pylori (*H. pylori*) is a spiral, flagellated, gram-negative bacteria, adapted to survive in the gastric lumen [1]. *H. pylori* is a bacterium that causes widespread infection, affecting over 50% of the world's population, but 80% of infected people are asymptomatic and more common in developing countries [2].

Megaloblastic anemia can result from impaired DNA synthesis resulting from vitamin B_{12} (cobalamin) and folic acid deficiency. Microorganisms synthesize vitamin B_{12}, that is primarily found in low concentration levels in meals with an animal source,

IntechOpen

humans cannot synthesize vitamin B_{12}. Early detection of vitamin B_{12} deficiency and rapid treatment of is important, since it is a reversible cause of demyelinated nervous system and bone marrow failure [3]. infection with *H. pylori* causes gastritis and it is associated with the progress of micronutrient deficiencies, peptic ulcer, gastric carcinoma [4].

Thyroid gland is one of the crucial organs in the human body that produces basic hormones: triiodothyronine (T3) and tetra-iodothyroxine (T4) which have an essential part in control of metabolic functions, development and growth. Thyroid dysfunction affecting various vital activities; those subsequent from hypo or hyper thyroid gland action leading to increase or decrease thyroid hormones T3 and T4 [5].

Hashimoto's thyroiditis (HT) is the most widely autoimmune thyroid disorders as one of most complications of thyroid dysfunctions. Autoimmune diseases occur when the immune system begins to attack its own self-antigens, so, that the characteristic feature of autoimmune thyroid disease is the presence of autoantibodies against thyroid antigens. Such diseases are triggered by factors including infectious agents, just like as infection with *H. pylori* [6, 7]. Luther et al. (2010) found that a high prevalence of people who have been diagnosed as thyroid patients were also infected with *H. pylori* which means that these bacteria play a critical part in the pathogenesis of such illnesses. *H. pylori* is one of the most well-known bacterial pathogens that infect human around the worldwide, which acquired in the early childhood and is carried throughout a lifetime if not treated with antimicrobial agents [8].

The present work sought to investigates the changes in vitamin B12, iron, thyroid hormones, thyroid autoantibodies and hematological indices levels in patients suffering from *H. pylori* infection.

2. *H. pylori*

2.1 General characteristics

H. pylori is considered to be as one of the furthermost common pathogenic bacteria that colonizes human stomach, varying from 70% in developing countries and less than 40% in the developed countries [9]. *H. pylori* is the main causative agent of gastritis and responsible for development of adenocarcinoma by stimulating cell proliferation and induces apoptosis [10]. *H. pylori* is a Gram- negative spiral bacteria measuring 2–4 μm in length, 0.5–1 μm in width and has 2–6 sheathed flagella 3 μm in length (Guo et al., 2011). *H. pylori* growth at optimal rang of: temperature 34-40C°, pH 5.5–8.0 but can survive at pH 4 and the key feature of *H. pylori* its microaerophilicity. Growth at optimal level of: 2–5% oxygen, 5–10% carbon dioxide and 85% nitrogen [11].

H. pylori is microaerophilic bacterium, requires lower oxygen concentrations than other bacteria to exist. It has a hydrogenase that may be utilized to generate energy by oxidizing the molecular hydrogen (H_2) produced by intestinal bacteria, and it can generates urease, catalase, and oxidase [12]. These bacteria survive in the stomach for a long time without any indications in most of the infected people. In order to inhabit the stomach, *H. pylori* must survive in acidic pH, its persistence be influenced by the production of urease enzyme, in addition to this enzyme these pathogenic bacteria produce other enzymes which damage of host epithelial cells such as catalase, protease and phospholipase. *H. pylori* are vital for colonizing the stomach and make it possible for it to pass readily through the mucous layer [13].

2.2 *H. pylori* classification

H. pylori genus is a *Helicobacteraceae* family member and *Campylobacterales* order of proteobacteria. The digestive tracts of both humans and animals naturally contain the genus *Helicobacter*, which has more than 20 identified species and several more that are waiting proper classification [14].

2.3 Prevalence of *H. pylori* infection

H. pylori infection prevalence rates vary by age, place of origin, and socioeconomic position. Worldwide, *H. pylori* infection affects 50% of the population [15]. According to reports, up to 80% of people in undeveloped countries are infected with *H. pylori*. In Texas, the incidence of *H. pylori* among youngsters is 12.2%, whereas in India, it is 55.9% among people aged 11–16. [15, 16], and in northern Jordan is 82% [17] and in Gaza strip is (72.2%) [18].

2.4 Mode of transmission

2.4.1 Person-person route

Humans have been identified as a major *H. pylori* reservoir [19]. Person to-person contact is believed to be the primary route of transmission in developed and developing countries. Close personal relationships, especially those inside the family, between parents and children, siblings and siblings, and spouses and spouses, has been consistently verified as a major factor of transmission [20].

2.4.2 Oral-oral route

Using a polymerase chain reaction, *H. pylori* DNA has been found in the saliva of people who tested positive [21]. Additionally, *H. pylori* bacteria have been effectively found in infected dental plaque. However, isolation has not always been effective, possibly due to *H. pylori's* transitory existence in the buccal cavity or low detection capabilities brought on by the co-existence of several other microorganisms.

2.4.3 Fecal-oral route

Fecal-oral is the main route of *H. pylori* transmission, *H. pylori* has been identified in human feces by culture and by PCR of its DNA. [22] Nevertheless, this has not been replicated by other researchers [23]. These findings provided evidence of the potential contribution of *H. pylori* fecal shedding into the environment.

2.4.4 Iatrogenic transmission

Endoscopes frequently utilized for upper gastrointestinal procedures, because they aren't properly disinfected in between procedures, could be the cause of an iatrogenic infection [24].

2.4.5 Mechanisms of infection

Most *H. pylori* are located in the gastric mucosa of the stomach; however, a few are also observed adherent to the gastric mucosal epithelium. The bacteria are well suited to survive in the harsh conditions of the stomach, where very few others organisms can. Despite the fact that *H. pylori* is thought of as an extracellular bacteria, there is evidence that the bacteria have a method of intracellular invasion [25]. The human stomach is colonized by *H. pylori*, and about 50% of the worldwide people is colonized by it. Its gastric mucosa infection has been related to a variety of upper gastrointestinal tract illnesses, including chronic gastritis, peptic ulcer, stomach cancer and mucosa-associated lymphoid tissue lymphoma [26]. *H. pylori* typically results in an asymptomatic stomach infection, and documented side effects of this infection include chronic gastritis, peptic ulcer disease, and atrophic gastritis. Most infected individuals remain asymptomatic despite the fact that the infection almost always results in stomach inflammation, whereas a small percentage of people develop atrophic gastritis [27]. During its progression, the disease can have several manifestations including acute gastritis, chronic atrophic gastritis, intestinal metaplasia, dysplasia, growth failure, malnutrition and finally cancer [28]. *H pylori* is the major cause of histologic gastritis and also plays an important role in the development of peptic ulcers, gastric carcinoma, and primary gastric B-cell lymphoma [29].

The etiology of atrophic gastritis and gastric cancer has been rewritten since the detection of *H. pylori* during the 1980s. *H. pylori* infection, which typically develops in early childhood and lasts a lifetime if untreated, is now recognized as the primary cause of atrophic gastritis [27]. One severe consequence of atrophic gastritis is the malabsorption of cobalamin (vitamin B_{12}), which is frequent in the elderly due to hypo- or achlorhydria with subsequent bacterial overgrowth, and reduced production and secretion of intrinsic factor. Carmel et al., hypothesized that *H. pylori* infection may be crucial in the decline in acid production, the reduction in intrinsic factor secretion, and the subsequent emergence of vitamin B_{12} insufficiency [30]. *H. pylori* inhabiting the whole gastric epithelial and has a significant urease activity that results in the creation of ammonia to protect itself against the acidity of the stomach. It also produces other enzymes, including glycosulfatase and phospholipase A2 and C, which are associated with the development of stomach mucosal injury [31]. *H. pylori* induces an inflammatory response through the gastric epithelium, with production of pro-inflammatory cytokines, such as interleukin 1β and interleukin 8. Some *H. pylori* genotypes, especially those vacuolating toxin A (Vac-A) and cytotoxin-associated gene A (Cag-A) positive, are associated with greater pathogenicity and more severe sickness. Cag-A positive strains cause the stomach mucosa to react more violently to inflammation and produce more pro-inflammatory cytokines. Even while it only phenotypically manifests in 60% of *H. pylori* strains, the VacA gene, which causes the vacuolization and death of gastric epithelial cells, is genetically expressed in all of them [32]. Gastritis, including atrophic and non-atrophic gastritis, and peptic ulcers, are etiologically linked to *H. pylori* (especially duodenal ulcer). The primary gastric B-cell lymphoma (also known as mucosa-associated-lymphatic-tissue or MALT-lymphoma) and stomach adenocarcinoma have a strong correlation with *H. pylori*. *H. pylori* has been therefore classified by IARC/WHO as "group 1 carcinogen" [33].

2.5 Diagnosis of *H. pylori* infection

Infections are typically diagnosed by looking for dyspeptic symptoms and performing tests that may reveal *H. pylori* infection [34]. The diagnostic tools for *H. pylori* are serology, rapid urease test (RUT), urea breath test (UBT), endoscopy and biopsy/

histopathology, PCR, for DNA of *H. pylori* and *H. pylori* stool antigen (HpSA). The simplest test of *H. pylori* is serologic, including the assessment of specific IgG level in serum [27, 35].

3. Anemia

3.1 Definition of anemia

Anemia is the most common blood disorder is characterized by a decrease in the number of red blood cells or a less-than-normal quantity of hemoglobin in the blood. The most widely used standards of anemia are those set by the World Health Organization, which identify hemoglobin levels of less below 12 g/dL for women and bellow 13 g/dL for males [36]. Globally, the most prevalent type of anemia was iron deficiency. It is a major public health issue that affects both advanced and developing societies, having a significant negative impact on people's health as well as social and economic development.

3.2 Common causes of anemia

Anemia from active bleeding; Heavy menstrual bleeding or, wounds and gastrointestinal ulcers or cancers [37, 38]. *Iron deficiency anemia;* Inadequate food intake, poor health and improper care [39]. *Anemia of chronic disease;* Long-term medical condition such as a chronic infection or a cancer [40]. *Anemia related to kidney disease*; Diminish production of renal erythropoietin which in turn diminishes the production of RBC [41]. *Anemia related to pregnancy*; Water weight gain during pregnancy dilutes the blood, which may be reflected as anemia [42]. *Anemia related to poor nutrition*; Deficiency of vitamins and minerals required to make RBC [42]. *Pernicious anemia*; A problem in the stomach or the intestines leading to poor absorption of vitamin B_{12} [43]. *Sickle cell anemia*; Is due to a point mutation in the β globin gene, resulting in the creation of abnormal hemoglobin molecules with a hydrophobic motif that is exposed in its deoxygenated state [44]. *Hemolytic anemia*; hemolysis-related anemia, which is caused by the abnormal breakdown of RBC, blood vessels, and extravascular locations throughout the body [45]. *Thalassemia*; This is another group of hereditary anemia of hemoglobin related causes. It varies in severity from mild thalassemia minor to severe thalassemia major [46]. *A plastic anemia*; Occasionally some viral infections may severely affect the bone marrow and significantly diminish production of all blood cells chemotherapy (cancer medications) and some other medications may pose the same problems and radiation [47].

3.3 Iron deficiency anemia

3.3.1 Definition

Iron deficiency anemia (IDA) is A decrease in overall hemoglobin concentration caused on by a deficiency of iron required for maintaining normal physiologic processes. Iron deficiency anemia results from inadequate iron absorption to a accommodate an increase in requirements attributable to growth or arising from a prolonged negative iron balance, one of these conditions causes a reduction in iron storage as indicated by blood ferritin levels or bone marrow iron content [48].

3.3.2 Causes

Iron-deficiency anemia may develop from a variety of conditions, including stomach ulcers, ulcerative colitis, piles, and colon cancer, which can all induce gut bleeding and result in anemia. Anemia can be brought on by bleeding brought on by kidney or bladder illness. Anemia caused by iron deficiency can be brought on by a number of illnesses, including cancer and rheumatoid arthritis. Iron deficiency anemia is correlated with long-term aspirin use [49].

3.3.3 Diagnosis of iron deficiency anemia

Iron deficiency anemia were diagnosed by the first result on a regular complete blood count is typically low hemoglobin in the context of a lowered MCV, and the ferritin level was below 1010 ng/dl [50].

3.3.4 Pathophysiology of iron deficiency by H. pylori

Common symptoms of IDA include: breathlessness, tiredness, dizziness, tachycardia, headache and paleness [51]. The pathophysiologic mechanisms by which *H. pylori* is associated with the development of ID and ID anemia are not fully understood. It is still not known why some patients manifest this association and why in other patients it is not present, or there are other associations; or why some of the infections are asymptomatic [15]. Over the past decade, it has been linked *H. pylori* and ID development with a recently discovered hormone called hepcidin [52]. This hormone is produced in the liver and regulates iron metabolism in enterocytes and releases stored iron from macrophages of the reticuloendothelial system [53]. Hepcidin increases following *H. pylori* infection and acts as an acute phase reactant in reaction to the inflammation created in the gastric mucosa, culminating in a condition characterized as chronic illness or inflammatory anemia [54]. According to preliminary research, serum levels of hepcidin were raised in *H. pylori*-infected patients but returned to normal after the infection was eradicated, allowing the iron to be absorbed by enterocytes and freed from reticuloendothelial system macrophages, where it had been trapped [55]. Other possible causes of iron imbalance in patients infected with *H. pylori* are chronic gastritis, which occurs in all individuals infected with *H. pylori* [15]. This can cause bleeding when it becomes erosive gastritis, especially in patients with active bleeding peptic ulcers [56] and in patients who chronically ingest non-steroidal anti-inflammatory drug including aspirin [43].

3.4 Vitamin B_{12}

3.4.1 Definition and structure

Vitamin B_{12} or cyanocobalamin is relatively large and complex water-soluble vitamin. The molecular weight of vitamin B_{12} is equal to 1355.4 [57]. All cobalamins that may be physiologically active are represented by vitamin B12. The name "cobalamin" is used to describe a class of cobalt-containing substances known as corrinoids, each of which has a lower axial ligand that contains a cobalt-coordinated nucleotide (5,6-dimethylbenzimidazole as a base. Cyanocobalamin, which is used in most supplements, is readily converted to the coenzyme forms of cobalamin (methylcobalamin and 5- deoxyadenosylcobalamin) in the human body [58]. The partial structures of vitamin B_{12} compounds show only those portions of the molecule that differ from vitamin B_{12} 1: 5-deoxyadenosylcobalamin; 2,'methylcobalamin; 3, hydroxocobalamin; 4, sulfitocobalamin; 5, cyanocobalamin or vitamin B_{12} [57].

3.4.2 Sources of vitamin B_{12}

Vitamin B_{12} is synthesized only in certain bacteria [59]. In the natural food chain system, more predatory organisms have larger concentrations of vitamin B_{12} that bacteria produce. The main dietary sources of vitamin B_{12} are thought to be animal foods (meat, milk, eggs, fish, and shellfish) rather than plant foods [58]. Some plant foods, such as edible algae or blue-green algae (cyanobacteria), however, contain large amounts of vitamin B_{12}. Vitamin B_{12} compounds in algae appear to be inactive in mammals [60]. Foods contain various vitamin B_{12} compounds with different upper ligands; methylcobalamin and 5-deoxyadenosylcobalamin function, respectively, as coenzymes of methionine synthase (EC 2.1.1.13), which is involved in methionine biosynthesis and of methylmolonyl- CoA mutase (EC 5.4.99.2), which is involved in amino acid and odd-chain fatty acid metabolism in mammalian cells [61]. Humans have a complex process for gastrointestinal absorption of dietary vitamin B_{12} [62]. The recommended dietary allowance of vitamin B_{12} for adults is set at 2.4 μg/day in the United States and Japan; however, daily body loss of the vitamin is estimated to be between 2 and 5 μg/day [63]. According to a study by Bor et al., in 2006, a daily consumption of 6 μg of vitamin B12 is sufficient to maintain a stable level of serum vitamin B_{12} and vitamin B_{12}-related metabolic indicators [64].

3.4.3 Vitamin B_{12} functions

Cobalamin, or vitamin B_{12}, comes in a variety of forms, such as cyano-, methyl-, deoxyadenosyl-, and hydroxy-cobalamin. Food contains small amounts of the cyano form, which would be utilized in supplements. The other forms of cobalamin can be changed into the methyl- or 5-deoxyadenosyl forms that seem to be necessary as cofactors for L-methyl-malonyl-CoA mutase and methionine synthase. For the formation of purines and pyrimidines, methionine synthase is necessary. The reaction, in which the methyl group of methyltetrahydrofolate is transferred to homocysteine to generate methionine and tetrahydrofolate, requires folate as a co-factor and also depends on methylcobalamin. Megaloblastic anemia develops as a result of a vitamin B12 shortage and the disruption of the process that causes RBCs to mature. Megaloblastic anemia is also brought on by a folate deficit, which is unrelated to vitamin B12 [65]. Methylmalonyl CoA mutase changes methylmalonyl CoA into succinyl CoA, and it needs the cofactor 5-deoxyadenosylcobalamin to do so. The neurological consequences of vitamin B12 deficiency are assumed to be caused by a flaw in this process and the accompanying buildup of methylmalonyl CoA [65].

3.4.4 Deficiency of vitamin B_{12}

Vitamin B_{12} deficiency is usually caused by the malabsorption of vitamin B_{12} although dietary inadequacy is common in the elderly, vegans or ovo-lacto vegetarians with poor diets. Other contributing factors include insufficient intrinsic factor synthesis, atrophic gastritis, disease-related disruption of vitamin B12 absorption in the ileum, bacterial overgrowth, resection, drug-nutrient interactions, and other less prevalent genetic abnormalities [66]. Pernicious anemia is the end stage of an auto-immune gastritis and results in the loss of synthesis of IF. It is this loss of IF that causes vitamin B_{12} deficiency and if untreated, megaloblastic anemia and neurological complications develop [66].

3.4.5 Mechanism of vitamin B_{12} deficiency

A mechanism that has been proposed to explain this association is that the action of *H. pylori* decreases gastric acid secretions which leads to hypochlorhydria [67]. On the one hand, protein-bound vitamin B_{12} must be released by the action of gastric acid in the stomach, yet hypochlorhydria itself increases the bacteria of the stomach and intestines. These bacteria may in turn make use of the vitamin B_{12} themselves [68]. This mechanism is supported decreased vitamin B_{12} levels secondary to chronic use of PPIs [69]. In addition, it has been proposed that vitamin B_{12} deficiency is secondary to decreased production of intrinsic factor due to atrophic gastritis (pernicious anemia) which results from chronic *H. pylori* infections [70]. However, one study has concluded that the association between *H. pylori* and vitamin B12 deficiency is independent of atrophic gastritis [71].

3.5 Thyroid hormones and autoantibodies

3.5.1 Thyroid hormones

The thyroid gland, which is shaped like a butterfly and is located at the base of the neck right behind the larynx, generates the essential hormones T4 and T3 [72]. Thyroid hormones are essential for numerous functions including: brain development, growth, fuel metabolism, reproduction, regulate body temperature and blood pressure [73]. TSH, which is made by the pituitary gland and regulates the production of T3 and T4, was responsible for controlling T3 and T4 levels. TSH production controlled by thyroid releasing hormone (TRH) produced by the hypothalamus [74]. This means that thyroid gland regulates its hormonal secretion with the aid of hypothalamus and the pituitary gland in a way that TRH is triggered pituitary to secrete TSH which in turn tells thyroid gland to capture iodine from the blood to synthesized and produced T4 and T3. Hypothalamus and pituitary gland decrease TRH and TSH when T4 is reach to a satisfactory level in circulation [75].

3.5.2 Thyroid autoantibodies

Auto-antibodies cause cellular damage and modify thyroid gland function. Sensitized T-lymphocytes and/or autoantibodies that attach to thyroid cell membranes result in cell lysis and inflammatory responses, causing cellular damage. Alterations in thyroid gland function result from the action of stimulating or blocking auto-antibodies on cell membrane receptors. TPO, Tg, and the TSH receptor are the three main thyroid auto-antigens involved in autoimmune thyroid disease (ATD). [75]. Thyroid peroxidase is the key enzyme catalyzing both the iodination and coupling reaction for the synthesis of thyroid hormone. It is membrane-bound and found in the cytoplasm of thyrocyte. It was earlier known as thyroid microsomal antigen. Anti-TPO autoantibodies are found in patients with autoimmune hypothyroidism and Graves' disease (GD). Together with Tg antibodies, these are the predominant antibodies in Hashimoto's thyroiditis. Anti-TPO antibodies are mainly of the IgG class with IgG1and IgG4 subclasses in excess [76].

Thyroglobulin made out of two identical subunits. It is discharged by the thyroid follicular cells into the follicular lumen and stored as the colloid. Each Tg molecule has around 100 tyrosine residues. These deposits were coupled to form the thyroid hormones T3 and T4. The sequence of human Tg has been determined [77]. Thyroglobulin autoantibodies are found in patients with lymphocytic thyroiditis and Graves' disease patients. They are polyclonal and mainly of IgG class with all four subclasses represented. TSH controls the cell surface expression of TPO and Tg altering the mRNA transcription of these two proteins. Both blocking and stimulating Autoantibodies are found in the sera of GD patients replicate these effects [78].

Our previous experimental results [79] indicated statistically significant positive correlation between TSH levels and anti TPO and anti Tg at baseline. Also, there were statistically significant negative correlations between fT3, fT4 levels and anti-TPO and anti-Tg. This result agrees with a previous study in which statistically significant positive correlations between TSH levels and anti TPO and anti-Tg were reported. Also these findings are in agreement with that obtained by [80]. Lin et al. (2014) who found elevated levels of both anti-Tg and anti-TPO in patients with radiation-induced hypothyroidism, in addition to positive correlation between TSH and anti-Tg and a negative correlation between fT4 and anti-TPO [80].

Hou et al. (2017) who observed reduction of thyroid autoantibodies in patients with GD and HT after pharmaceutical eradication of *H. pylori* infection [81]. *H. pylori* plays role in ATD pathogenesis. Genetic factors include thyroid specific genes and immune regulatory genes while none genetic factors include: smoking, stress, iodine intake, medication, pregnancy and bacterial and virus infection that have been implicated with etiology of ATD [82]. Strong correlation between IgG anti–*H. pylori* antibodies and thyroid auto-antibodies as well as the observation that eradication of *H. pylori* infection is followed by gradual decrease in the levels of thyroid auto-antibodies, supposed that *H. pylori* antigens might be involved in the development of autoimmuno atrophic thyroiditis or that autoimmuno function in this disease may increase the likelihood of *H. pylori* infection [83]. El-Eshmawy et al., (2011) who found that a correlation between *H. pylori* infection and the presence of autoantibodies against thyroid antigens, and highly significant prevalence of *H. pylori* infection in the ATD patients when compared with healthy individuals [84].

4. Conclusions

H. pylori appears to play a role in the onset of IDA and vitamin B_{12}. *H. pylori* patients had significant decreases in vitamin B_{12}, serum iron and hemoglobin levels. An insufficient response to the medication may be caused by *H. pylori* gastritis. A raise in *H. pylori* IgG, anti-TPO, anti-TG, and TSH levels and a decrease in fT4, fT3, and other hematological markers appear to before *H. pylori* treatment in hypothyroidism Palestinian females. Patients receiving triple therapy for *H. pylori* infection OAC may help patients feel better overall by restoring their vitamin B12, serum iron, and hemoglobin levels. In people with gastritis, vitamin B12 levels are highly associated with Hb and RBCs. As a result, it could be thought of as a helpful indicator for patients with anemia with gastritis. *H. pylori* is responsible for hypothyroid patients getting large doses of L-T4 poor response. However, these parameters were nearly improved by 14-day conventional triple treatment with omeprazole, amoxicillin, and clarithromycin. Routine testing of vitamin B_{12}, iron, ferritin and total iron binding capacity level and immunological thyroid alterations were recommended for *H. pylori* patients and gastroscopy confirmation of *H. pylori* infection.

Conflict of interest

The authors declare no conflict of interest.

Author details

Saleh Nazmy Mwafy*, Wesam Mohammad Afana and Asma'a Ali Hejaze
Faculty of Science, Department of Biology, Al Azhar University – Gaza, Gaza Strip, Palestine

*Address all correspondence to: smwafy@hotmail.com

References

[1] Calam J. *Discovery and bacteriology*. In: *Clinicians' Guide to Helicobacter pylori*. New York, NY: Springer; 1996. pp. 1-21

[2] Devrajani BR et al. Type 2 diabetes mellitus: A risk factor for *Helicobacter pylori* infection: A hospital based case-control study. International Journal of Diabetes in Developing Countries. 2010;**30**(1):22

[3] Stabler SP. Vitamin B12 deficiency. New England Journal of Medicine. 2013;**368**(2):149-160

[4] Rothenbacher D, Brenner H. Burden of *Helicobacter pylori* and *H. pylori*-related diseases in developed countries: Recent developments and future implications. Microbes and Infection. 2003;**5**(8):693-703

[5] Thiruvengadam S, Luthra P. Thyroid disorders in elderly: A comprehensive review. Disease-a-Month. 2021;**67**(11): 101223

[6] Swain M, Swain T, Mohanty BK. Autoimmune thyroid disorders—An update. Indian Journal of Clinical Biochemistry. 2005;**20**(1):9-17

[7] Lazúrová I, Benhatchi K. Autoimmune thyroid diseases and nonorgan-specific autoimmunity. Polskie Archiwum Medycyny Wewnetrznej. 2012;**122**:55-59

[8] Luther J et al. Association between *Helicobacter pylori* infection and inflammatory bowel disease: A meta-analysis and systematic review of the literature. Inflammatory Bowel Diseases. 2010;**16**(6):1077-1084

[9] Minov J et al. The impact of *Helicobacter pylori* infection on lung function and severity of bronchial hyperresponsiveness in subjects with allergic asthma. American Journal of Immunology. 2011;**7**(4):62-67

[10] Kim JM et al. Stimulation of dendritic cells with *Helicobacter pylori* vacuolating cytotoxin negatively regulates their maturation via the restoration of E2F1. Clinical & Experimental Immunology. 2011;**166**(1):34-45

[11] Guo C et al. Genotyping analysis of *Helicobacter pylori* using multiple-locus variable-number tandem-repeats analysis in five regions of China and Japan. BMC Microbiology. 2011;**11**(1):1-7

[12] Baldwin DN et al. Identification of *Helicobacter pylori* genes that contribute to stomach colonization. Infection and Immunity. 2007;**75**(2):1005-1016

[13] Ahmed S, Belayneh YM. *Helicobacter pylori* and duodenal ulcer: Systematic review of controversies in causation. Clinical and Experimental Gastroenterology. 2019;**12**:441

[14] Fox J. The non-*H pylori* helicobacters: Their expanding role in gastrointestinal and systemic diseases. Gut. 2002;**50**(2):273-283

[15] Correa P, Piazuelo MB. Natural history of *Helicobacter pylori* infection. Digestive and Liver Disease. 2008;**40**(7):490-496

[16] Mishra S et al. Prevalence of *Helicobacter pylori* in asymptomatic subjects—A nested PCR based study. Infection, Genetics and Evolution. 2008;**8**(6):815-819

[17] Bani-Hani KE, Hammouri SM. Prevalence of *Helicobacter pylori* in Northern Jordan. Endoscopy based

study. Saudi Medical Journal. 2001;**22**(10):843-847

[18] Mwafy SN, Afana WM. Hematological parameters, serum iron and vitamin B 12 levels in hospitalized Palestinian adult patients infected with *Helicobacter pylori*: A case–control study. Hematology, Transfusion and Cell Therapy. 2018;**40**:160-165

[19] Stefano K et al. *Helicobacter pylori*, transmission routes and recurrence of infection: State of the art. Acta Bio Medica: Atenei Parmensis. 2018;**89**(Suppl. 8):72

[20] Khalifa MM, Sharaf RR, Aziz RK. *Helicobacter pylori*: A poor man's gut pathogen? Gut Pathogens. 2010;**2**(1):1-12

[21] Leonardi M et al. Assessment of real-time PCR for *Helicobacter pylori* DNA detection in stool with co-infection of intestinal parasites: A comparative study of DNA extraction methods. BMC Microbiology. 2020;**20**(1):1-8

[22] Momtaz H et al. Study of *Helicobacter pylori* genotype status in saliva, dental plaques, stool and gastric biopsy samples. World Journal of Gastroenterology: WJG. 2012;**18**(17):2105

[23] van Zwet AA et al. Use of PCR with feces for detection of *Helicobacter pylori* infections in patients. Journal of Clinical Microbiology. 1994;**32**(5):1346-1348

[24] Brown LM. *Helicobacter pylori*: Epidemiology and routes of transmission. Epidemiologic Reviews. 2000;**22**(2):283-297

[25] Kusters JG, Van Vliet AH, Kuipers EJ. Pathogenesis of *Helicobacter pylori* infection. Clinical Microbiology Reviews. 2006;**19**(3):449-490

[26] Dunne C, Dolan B, Clyne M. Factors that mediate colonization of the human stomach by *Helicobacter pylori*. World Journal of Gastroenterology: WJG. 2014;**20**(19):5610

[27] Suerbaum S, Michetti P. *Helicobacter pylori* infection. New England Journal of Medicine. 2002;**347**(15):1175-1186

[28] Windle HJ, Kelleher D, Crabtree JE. Childhood *Helicobacter pylori* infection and growth impairment in developing countries: A vicious cycle? Pediatrics. 2007;**119**(3):e754-e759

[29] DIXON MF. *Helicobacter pylori* and peptic ulceration: Histopathological aspects. Journal of Gastroenterology and Hepatology. 1991;**6**(2):125-130

[30] Carmel R. Cobalamin, the stomach, and aging. The American Journal of Clinical Nutrition. 1997;**66**(4):750-759

[31] Dzierzanowska-Fangrat K, Dzierzanowska D. *Helicobacter pylori*: Microbiology and interactions with gastrointestinal microflora. Journal of Physiology and Pharmacology: An Official Journal of the Polish Physiological Society. 2006;**57**:5-14

[32] Yamaoka Y. Mechanisms of disease: *Helicobacter pylori* virulence factors. Nature Reviews Gastroenterology & Hepatology. 2010;**7**(11):629-641

[33] Pandey R et al. *Helicobacter pylori* and gastric cancer. Asian Pacific Journal of Cancer Prevention. 2010;**11**(3):583-588

[34] Stenström B, Mendis A, Marshall B. *Helicobacter pylori*: The latest in diagnosis and treatment. Australian Journal of General Practice. 2008;**37**(8):608

[35] Tiwari SK et al. Rapid diagnosis of *Helicobacter pylori* infection in dyspeptic patients using salivary secretion: A

non-invasive approach. Singapore Medical Journal. 2005;**46**(5):224-228

[36] Khusun H et al. World Health Organization hemoglobin cut-off points for the detection of anemia are valid for an Indonesian population. The Journal of Nutrition. 1999;**129**(9):1669-1674

[37] Dicato M, Plawny L, Diederich M. Anemia in cancer. Annals of Oncology. 2010;**21**:vii167-vii172

[38] Villanueva C et al. Transfusion strategies for acute upper gastrointestinal bleeding. New England Journal of Medicine. 2013;**368**(1):11-21

[39] Vieth JT, Lane DR. Anemia. Emergency Medicine Clinics. 2014;**32**(3): 613-628

[40] Guidi GC, Santonastaso CL. Advancements in anemias related to chronic conditions. Clinical Chemistry and Laboratory Medicine. 2010;**48**(9):1217-1226

[41] O'Mara NB. Anemia in patients with chronic kidney disease. Diabetes Spectrum. 2008;**21**(1):12-20

[42] Huret J-L, Dessen P, Bernheim A. Atlas of genetics and cytogenetics in oncology and haematology, year 2003. Nucleic Acids Research. 2003;**31**(1):272-274

[43] Song HJ et al. Cost effectiveness associated with *Helicobacter pylori* screening and eradication in patients taking nonsteroidal anti-inflammatory drugs and/or aspirin. Gut and Liver. 2013;**7**(2):182

[44] Malowany JI, Butany J. *Pathology of sickle cell disease*. *Seminars in Diagnostic Pathology*. 2012;**29**:49-55

[45] Means RT. Iron deficiency and iron deficiency anemia: Implications and impact in pregnancy, fetal development, and early childhood parameters. Nutrients. 2020;**12**(2):447

[46] Higgs DR, Engel JD, Stamatoyannopoulos G. Thalassaemia. The Lancet. 2012;**379**(9813):373-383

[47] Gupta V et al. Cytogenetic profile of aplastic anaemia in Indian children. The Indian Journal of Medical Research. 2013;**137**(3):502

[48] Baker RD, Greer FR, C.o. Nutrition, *diagnosis and prevention of iron deficiency and iron-deficiency anemia in infants and young children (0-3 years of age)*. Pediatrics. 2010;**126**(5):1040-1050

[49] Bayraktar UD, Bayraktar S. Treatment of iron deficiency anemia associated with gastrointestinal tract diseases. World Journal of Gastroenterology: WJG. 2010;**16**(22):2720

[50] Bermejo F, García-López S. A guide to diagnosis of iron deficiency and iron deficiency anemia in digestive diseases. World Journal of Gastroenterology: WJG. 2009;**15**(37):4638

[51] Zhu A, Kaneshiro M, Kaunitz JD. Evaluation and treatment of iron deficiency anemia: A gastroenterological perspective. Digestive Diseases and Sciences. 2010;**55**(3):548-559

[52] Park CH et al. Hepcidin, a urinary antimicrobial peptide synthesized in the liver. Journal of Biological Chemistry. 2001;**276**(11):7806-7810

[53] Kroot JJ et al. Hepcidin in human iron disorders: Diagnostic implications. Clinical Chemistry. 2011;**57**(12):1650-1669

[54] Cherian S et al. An insight into the relationships between hepcidin, anemia, infections and inflammatory cytokines

in pediatric refugees: A cross-sectional study. PLoS One. 2008;**3**(12):e4030

[55] Ozkasap S et al. The role of prohepcidin in anemia due to *Helicobacter pylori* infection. Pediatric Hematology and Oncology. 2013;**30**(5):425-431

[56] Kang JM et al. Risk factors for peptic ulcer bleeding in terms of *Helicobacter pylori*, NSAIDs, and antiplatelet agents. Scandinavian Journal of Gastroenterology. 2011;**46**(11):1295-1301

[57] Watanabe F. Vitamin B12 sources and bioavailability. Experimental Biology and Medicine. 2007;**232**(10):1266-1274

[58] Ball G. *Vitamin K*. In: *BioaVailability and Analysis of Vitamins in Foods*. Boston, MA: Springer; 1998. pp. 241-266

[59] Schneider Z, Stroinski A. Biosynthesis of vitamin B12. Comprehensive B. 1987;**12**:93-110

[60] Watanabe F et al. Characterization and bioavailability of vitamin B12-compounds from edible algae. Journal of Nutritional Science and Vitaminology. 2002;**48**(5):325-331

[61] Fenton WA et al. Purification and properties of methylmalonyl coenzyme A mutase from human liver. Archives of Biochemistry and Biophysics. 1982;**214**(2):815-823

[62] Russell-Jones GJ, Alpers DH. Vitamin B 12 transporters. Membrane Transporters as Drug Targets. 2002;**12**:493-520

[63] Yates AA, Schlicker SA, Suitor CW. Dietary reference intakes: the new basis for recommendations for calcium and related nutrients, B vitamins, and choline. Journal of the American Dietetic Association. 1998;**98**(6):699-706

[64] Bor MV et al. A daily intake of approximately 6 μg vitamin B-12 appears to saturate all the vitamin B-12–related variables in Danish postmenopausal women. The American Journal of Clinical Nutrition. 2006;**83**(1):52-58

[65] Gibson RS, Gibson RS. *Principles of Nutritional Assessment*. USA: Oxford University Press; 2005

[66] Park S, Johnson MA. What is an adequate dose of oral vitamin B12 in older people with poor vitamin B12 status? Nutrition Reviews. 2006;**64**(8):373-378

[67] Annibale B, Capurso G, Delle Fave G. Consequences of *Helicobacter pylori* infection on the absorption of micronutrients. Digestive and Liver Disease. 2002;**34**:S72-S77

[68] Baik H, Russell R. Vitamin B12 deficiency in the elderly. Annual Review of Nutrition. 1999;**19**:357

[69] Ito T, Jensen RT. Association of long-term proton pump inhibitor therapy with bone fractures and effects on absorption of calcium, vitamin B12, iron, and magnesium. Current Gastroenterology Reports. 2010;**12**(6):448-457

[70] Lahner E, Persechino S, Annibale B. Micronutrients (other than iron) and *Helicobacter pylori* infection: A systematic review. Helicobacter. 2012;**17**(1):1-15

[71] Serin E et al. Impact of *Helicobacter pylori* on the development of vitamin B12 deficiency in the absence of gastric atrophy. Helicobacter. 2002;**7**(6):337-341

[72] Mohmed MSA. Evaluation of Lipids Profile among Sudanese Patients with Hypothyroidism in Khartoum State. Master thesis on SUST Repository, Sudan

University of Science & Technology; 2018

[73] Sherwood L. *Human Physiology: From Cells to Systems*. Boston, MA: Cengage Learning; 2015

[74] Ferrara SJ, Bourdette D, Scanlan TS. Hypothalamic-pituitary-thyroid axis perturbations in male mice by CNS-penetrating thyromimetics. Endocrinology. 2018;**159**(7):2733-2740

[75] Ortiga-Carvalho TM et al. Hypothalamus-pituitary-thyroid axis. Comprehensive Physiology. 2011;**6**(3):1387-1428

[76] Kandi S, Rao P. *Anti-thyroid peroxidase antibodies: Its effect on thyroid gland and breast tissue*. Annals of Tropical Medicine & Public Health. 2012;**5**(1):1-3

[77] Gardner DG. Endocrine emergencies: Myxedema coma. Greenspan's Basic Clinical Endocrinology. 2007;**8**:868-870

[78] Iddah M, Macharia B. *Autoimmune thyroid disorders*. International Scholarly Research Notices. 2013;**2013**:1-9

[79] Mwafy S, Hejaze A. *Physiological Assessment of Hypothyroidism Females Infected with Helicobacter Pylori*. Master thesis on AUG Repository, Al Azhar University-Gaza; 2019

[80] Lin Z et al. Longitudinal study on the correlations of thyroid antibody and thyroid hormone levels after radiotherapy in patients with nasopharyngeal carcinoma with radiation-induced hypothyroidism. Head & Neck. 2014;**36**(2):171-175

[81] Hou Y et al. Meta-analysis of the correlation between *Helicobacter pylori* infection and autoimmune thyroid diseases. Oncotarget. 2017;**8**(70):115691

[82] Hamid ZA. The possible role of *Helicobacter pylori* infection in Hashimoto's thyroiditis. Journal of the Faculty of Medicine Baghdad. 2017;**59**(1):79-82

[83] Papamichael KX et al. Helicobacter pylori infection and endocrine disorders: Is there a link? World Journal of Gastroenterology: WJG. 2009;**15**(22):2701

[84] El-Eshmawy MM et al. *Helicobacter pylori* infection might be responsible for the interconnection between type 1 diabetes and autoimmune thyroiditis. Diabetology & Metabolic Syndrome. 2011;**3**(1):1-7

Chapter 6

Helicobacter Pylori Infection Correlates with Lower Prevalence and Subsequent Incidence of Crohn's Disease

Chenxiao Hu, Ting Lei, Natalie Tai, Yan Li, Xiujing Feng, Zhi Huang and Yun Lu

Abstract

According to some researchs, Crohn's disease (CD) and Ulcerative colitis (UC), two chronic inflammatory bowel illnesses, may be protected against *Helicobacter pylori* infection. Many case–control studies have revealed that individuals with CD and UC had lower *H. pylori* prevalence than healthy controls. However, whether or not *H. pylori* plays a protective role in the development of Crohn's disease is debatable. CD was more common in *H. pylori*-negative individuals than in *H. pylori*-positive patients. After eradication of *H. pylori*, the CD was more common in the *H. pylori*-negative group than in the *H. pylori*-positive group over the previous research follow-up period. Although it has been strongly indicated in previous studies that *H. pylori* infection plays a significant role and triggers autoimmune reactions and may be implicated in the pathogenesis of autoimmune diseases, the role of *H. pylori* in inflammatory bowel disease, including Crohn's disease, is unclear.

Keywords: *Helicobacter pylori*, Crohn's disease, immune cells, cytokines, Cronh's Disease and *H. pylori* correlation

1. Introduction

Crohn's disease (CD) is an inflammatory disease that could cause chronic inflammation throughout the gastrointestinal tract without a definite etiology [1]. Even though the incidence of CD has been increasing for several decades worldwide, it is more common in northern Europe and the United States compared to other areas, including southern Europe [2]. In addition to the primary contributor to the disease, which is the genetic predisposition, there is a growing body of evidence to support the concept that environmental variables, in particular the gut flora and antigens, are also involved in the development of Crohn's disease (CD). Several different infections have been proposed as potential causes of CD without solid evidence supporting these hypotheses. There is an unmet need to investigate the role of bacteria during CD development. Helicobacter pylori (*H. pylori*) is a type of bacteria that could cause ulcers in the stomach. Although it has been strongly indicated in previous studies that

H. pylori infection plays a significant role and triggers autoimmune reactions and may be implicated in the pathogenesis of autoimmune diseases, the role of *H. pylori* in inflammatory bowel disease (IBD), including Crohn's disease, is unclear [3].

H. pylori is a stain of Gram-negative bacteria that is very infectious and found in the mucosa of the human stomach. Chronic *H. pylori* infection is quite common. It is estimated that roughly 20 percent of Danish patients diagnosed with dyspepsia are infected with *H. pylori* [4]. Most cases of *H. pylori* infection occur in children and young adults [5]. Inadequate sanitation and poor socioeconomic standards have been reported as factors that correlate the increased risk of *H. pylori* infection, which is prevalent in certain countries such as India, China, and Brazil, where the incidence of *H. pylori* infection is considered over 50 percent [6]. Living quality and sanity go hand in hand with the development of the economy, which may explain why the prevalence of *H. pylori* infection has significantly decreased as the western style civilization grown grow. A persistent *H. pylori* infection is a significant factor for the development of chronic gastritis, peptic ulcer disease, and stomach cancer. Oddly, while the incidence of *H. pylori* infection has been going down, the number of people developing chronic inflammatory conditions including Crohn's disease is going up for no apparent reason [7]. This observation has given rise to the hypothesis that *H. pylori* infection may have host-protective role.

2. Epidemiological correlation between CD and *H. pylori*

H. pylori caused active infection is responsible for the prolonged inflammation of the colon and cecum that are seen in immunocompromised rodents [8–11]. However, the findings from patients were difficult to interpret. The intestinal mucosa of the majority of patients did not contain Helicobacter, or the presence of *H. pylori* was only discovered in a minority of those individuals [12–16]. In addition, results from meta-analysis revealed that *H. pylori* infection plays a protective role CD from an etiology point of view [10, 17–19]; however, the heterogeneity among the studies that were included in the meta-analysis and the possibility of publication bias limit the confidence that could be placed in these findings. Furthermore, it is still controversial whether *H. pylori* serves a protective role in the development of CD, a persistent inflammatory condition of gastrointestinal tract [18, 20]. As shown by the results, having *H. pylori* infection was associated with a lower risk of Crohn's disease (CD), and this correlation remains even after potential confounding factors such as socio-economic status were taken into account (**Table 1**) [6, 10, 19, 21–30]. On the other hand, it was revealed in other studies that the presence of an *H. pylori* infection was associated with an increased frequency of CD [18, 31, 32].

H. pylori infection and the prevalence of Crohn's disease, ulcerative colitis, and celiac disease also been investigated in a cohort of more than 50,000 Danish citizens who successively underwent a first-time urea breath test [33]. Although the previous research has shown that there is a correlation between *H. pylori* infection and IBD, the results have been inconsistent [33, 34]. The occurrences of CD, UC were used as part of a follow-up checklist in order to determine whether or not the possible protective benefits of *H. pylori* lingered after the bacteria has probably been eradicated.

A number of hypotheses have been proposed to explain this discovery. For instance, if patients with Crohn's disease received antibiotics prior to an *H. pylori* eradicating *H. pylori*, the rate of *H. pylori* infections in Crohn's disease patients would be smaller [33, 35–37]. This would lead to a reduction in the prevalence of *H. pylori*

Author	Pooled RR/OR	95% CI	p-Value
Yue et al. [21]	0.63	0.49–0.81	< 0.001
Luther et al. [22]	0.6	0.40–0.72	NR
Wu et al. [10]	0.43	0.37–0.50	< 0.001
Wang et al. [23]	0.41	0.32–0.53	< 0.001
Hesamaddin et al. [24]	0.40	0.33–0.49	< 0.001
Rokkas et al. [19]	0.38	0.31–0.47	< 0.001
Castañorodríguez et al. [25]	0.38	0.31–0.47	< 0.001
Ding et al. [26]	0.236	0.14–0.39	< 0.001

Table 1.
Helicobacter pylori infection rates in patients with CD.

infections in patients with CD. It is possible that *H. pylori* is just a proxy marker for exposure to an environment that protects against Crohn's disease. Alternatively, it may be a case of selection biases where patients seeing doctor regularly get tested for *H. pylori* more often than those patients seeing doctors for a cause [38]. There are various potential sources of bias and confounding variables, including the fact that individuals with Crohn's disease may have received other medical treatments that have an effect on *H. pylori*, or the fact that publishing biases may have distorted the findings [35, 39].

Various researches included the ecological epidemiology studies in order to tackle the issue of overcoming biases and confounding in their researches. Information regarding the prevalence and incidence of CD was combined with geographically and temporally matched studies of the prevalence of *H. pylori* [2, 3, 16, 17, 30, 39]. Shah et al. also expanded that epidemiology study strategy and conduct an in-depth analysis of the published researches on the epidemiology of Crohn's disease from 1990 to 2016, comparing the findings of this research with findings on the incidence of *H. pylori* infection. A combined data set included 22 incidence and 19 prevalence data pairs for Crohn's disease and *H. pylori* derived from 13 different countries was included [35, 40]. However, there are still a number of possible risks associated with the research. There is a possibility that the presence of *H. pylori* is not the sole factor that differentiates the non-exposed group from the group that has been exposed to *H. pylori*. Nevertheless, antibiotics may have been administered in an inconsistent manner, which may had an impact on the outcomes [41, 42]. During the time period between 1990 and 2016, these nations may have seen the most significant shifts in both the incidence and prevalence of CD, as well as the prevalence of *H. pylori*. The incidence of Crohn's disease is reduced in proportion to the percentage of the population that is infected with *H. pylori* [7, 15, 32, 33, 35].

3. Molecular mechanisms

A few different immunological mechanisms that are responsible for the possible negative correlation between *H. pylori* infection and IBD have been proposed. First, it was demonstrated that immune cell activation was suppressed by *H. pylori* DNA, including dendritic cells, macrophages, and other types of immune cells, which in turn reduced the severity of the colitis [43–45]. Other possible mechanisms by which gastric mucosa is protected by *H. pylori* infection from *S. typhimurium*-induced inflammation include the suppression of the inflammatory T helper 1/17 (Th1/17) response in the lower GI Tract. This has been found in mice, so was the increased production of the anti-inflammatory interleukin-10 (IL-10) in mesenteric lymph nodes [46, 47]. Infection with *H. pylori* may be associated with the presentation of microbiota in the gut. The presence of mutations in genes that are known to be associated with CD provided evidence that microbiota play a part in the pathogenesis of the illness. This might be accomplished by a change in the immune response, mucosal permeability, or the metabolic products of microbes [48–52]. Antibiotics and probiotics are two examples treatments targeting bacteria, and there has been a recent increase of the use of both approaches. Stomach mucosal infection caused by *H. pylori* has been shown to have an effect on the intestinal microbiota, resulting in a considerable decrease in gut inflammation. Treg cell activation is of the highest significance in this respect because Treg cells inhibit inflammatory and immunological responses to gut bacteria, perhaps by secreting anti-inflammatory and immunosuppressive cytokines [53–56]. This hypothesis helps to explain why the immune system tolerates a wide variety of "non-self" gut bacteria, despite their location on the mucosal surface of the digestive tract. It has been shown that infection with *H. pylori* increases the number of regulatory T cells in the mucosa of the stomach and in the peripheral circulation [54]. This infection also alters the actions of these cells, perhaps by affecting the expression of certain receptors. *H. pylori* modifies the host immune response to change the inflammatory Th1/17 pattern. This is accomplished by upregulating Foxp3, a marker of regulatory T cells, in the gastric mucosa. By inhibiting protective immunological response, regulatory T cells (also known as Treg cells) maintain a constant level of *H. pylori* colonization [57, 58]. Additionally, mucosal modifications that impede stomach colonization by *H. pylori* and/or its spontaneous elimination in response to CD therapy, particularly 5-aminosalicylic acid treatment, may account for the decreased incidence of *H. pylori* infection in CD patients [9, 59, 60].

Probiotics may be useful to reduce intestinal inflammation if they are administered to reestablish a healthy balance in the microbiota of the gut and/or to reset the immunological systems that have been dysregulated [19]. The anti-inflammatory and immune-modulatory effects of probiotics help decrease inflammation by inhibiting the production of pro-inflammatory cytokines and enhancing the production of anti-inflammatory cytokines. This is how probiotics work to reduce inflammation. There have been conflicting reports on using probiotics in terms of efficacy as part of a therapeutic strategy to eradicate *H. pylori*. In a number of clinical studies, the standard triple therapy for *H. pylori* was supplemented with adjuvant medications (such as lactoferrin and probiotics), trying to lower the risks of adverse side effects and raising the change of complete eradication [9, 35, 39, 50, 54]. The addition of lactoferrin or probiotics to the triple therapy did not result in an increase in the rate of *H. pylori* eradication; however, it did result in a reduction in epigastric pain, vomiting, and diarrhea, indicating a less degree of inflammation [53, 57]. This paradox may be caused antibiotic resistance, as well as the difference in treatment regimens used by different organizations.

The toxic strains of *H. pylori* are the most common cause of infection in people with CD. On the basis of the results of other studies demonstrating a higher incidence of Helicobacteraceae in patients with CD, it has been hypothesized that Helicobacteraceae may play a role in the etiology of CD, and that various strains of *H. pylori* may be able to adapt to colonize extra-gastric regions [61–64]. These hypotheses are based on the observation that CD patients have a higher prevalence of Helicobacteraceae. Additionally, it was shown that CD patients who exhibited a UC-like phenotype had higher prevalence rates of *H. pylori* in their stomachs [61, 64]. Because of the *H. pylori*-induced immune activation, there is a good chance that interleukin-12 (IL-12) and the Th1 immune response will be elevated [65, 66]. CD is an example of a Th1-related sickness, and TNF and IL-2 are two examples of Th1 cytokines that contribute to the development of the disease [66]. Infection with *H. pylori* promotes inflammation of the gut epithelium, which then secretes IL-8, attracting neutrophils that are involved in the pathogenesis of IBD [67, 68].

The elimination of *H. pylori* with the use of clarithromycin and/or proton pump inhibitors (PPIs) has been related to a decrease in Th1 factors, which may provide some degree of protection against CD [69, 70]. Nevertheless, no epidemiological data is available so far to support this idea. It has been shown that the common antibiotic clarithromycin has anti-inflammatory and immunomodulatory effects. These effects include a large decrease in the release and gene expression of Th1 factors and a smaller reduction in the synthesis of Th2 factors [71]. However, in other studies, it was shown that clarithromycin, but not amoxicillin, is able to reduce the levels of immunological components indicative of Th1, Th2, and Th17 [72–74]. Patients with steroid-sensitive asthma showed a decrease in Th2 factors after taking clarithromycin, whereas those with "infection-induced" steroid-resistant asthma showed a decrease in Th1/Th17 factors [72, 75]. In a randomized clinical trial that was controlled with a placebo, researchers found that the antibiotic clarithromycin was effective in treating persons with active CD for 1 month [76], possibly due to bacterial resistance. Because of the potential of PPIs to lower the amount of acid produced by the stomach, microbial growth in the upper GI tract may considerably increase. PPIs, on the other hand, inhibit the membrane H^+/-ATPase of some gut microorganisms, which results in bacteriostatic and even bactericidal effects. Omeprazole has been shown to provide complete relief from UC symptoms in as little as 5 days. Lansoprazole may be beneficial in the treatment of IBD, including CD, by inhibiting the synthesis of specific proinflammatory cytokines in macrophages. *In vitro* research result revealed that the addition of lansoprazole to the culture media led to a decrease in the production of inflammatory cytokines (TNF- and IL-1) [77], which were produced by monocytes from peripheral blood. Because of their anti-inflammatory and immunomodulatory nature, clarithromycin and PPIs have been proposed as potential preventative approaches for CD; however, the epidemiological data to support this hypothesis is inadequate.

Putting aside any and all objections, the current research is a significant evidence that lends credence to the idea that the occurrences of *H. pylori* and CD have an negative association. More and more research results with consistent finding on the relationship between *H. pylori* infection and the CD development have been published. It has been suggested that *H. pylori* induce the development of regulatory T cells and impairs dendritic cell maturation, consequently resulting in a tolerogenic phenotype, which is a part of the mechanisms that *H. pylori* utilize to avoid host immune reactions.

Recent research results suggest that the processes that are responsible for the association may be more convoluted than previously thought. This is due to the fact that variables other than *H. pylori* infection influences the progression of CD. The findings of Shah et al. suggest that *H. pylori* may "serve as a signal for other gastrointestinal illnesses," which would provide some protection against CD [40]. It is noted in this study that the microbiota in the upper gastrointestinal tract differ among individuals who are positive for *H. pylori* from individuals who are negative for the infection. Following the elimination of *H. pylori*, the changes of microbiota was found. Because it is considered that the gastrointestinal microbiota has a significant contribution to the development of CD, it is possible that a change in the components of the microbiota might change a person's vulnerability to CD. Since the relationship is clear, future research needs to focus more on the mechanisms that contribute to *H. pylori* infection, particularly in children. Another hotspot in the field would be the investigations focused on concomitant factors to *H. pylori* infection, such as alterations in the gut microbiota, which may potentially impact the etiology of Crohn's disease. A decision of the eradication of *H. pylori* in asymptomatic persons, in particular in patients with established Crohn's disease, should eventually be made based on the data collected from this type of researches.

4. Conclusion

Researchers have concluded that *H. pylori* should be classified as a suppress factor since patients with infections may have a reduced prevalence and subsequent incidence of CD. The Kyoto global agreement recommends eradicating *H. pylori* of each afflicted unless there are compelling reasons not to. This is because *H. pylori* may be associated with gastritis, which has been linked to an increased risk of developing stomach cancer. Despite the high infection incidence and the enormous amounts of antibiotics used, eradication of H. pylori has not been proven by various country recommendations. Unfortunately, epidemiologists specializing in *H. pylori control* paid little attention to the total impacts except for increased CD. *H. pylori* has an immunological tolerance mechanism, which allows it to stay in the mucosa while also the induced tolerogenic Th cells, immunosuppressive Tregs and cytokines are maintaining the critical systemic immune homeostasis. Consequently, the eradication of *H. pylori* with antibiotics is known to have greatly altered the microenvironment of gut bacteria. From the current review, this strategy has an indirect dramatic effect on immunological homeostasis, which may provide the potential risk of CD. The risk of gastric cancer in H. pylori-infected may not be calculated precisely, also the precise assessment of the risk of CD after *H. pylori* eradication is hard to be predicted and evaluated either. Therefore, the decreased prevalence and subsequent incidence of CD demonstrated the critical need for improved and individualized treatments for *H. pylori* infection.

Author details

Chenxiao Hu[1†], Ting Lei[2†], Natalie Tai[3], Yan Li[4], Xiujing Feng[4], Zhi Huang[5*†] and Yun Lu[6*†]

1 The Information Center, The 1st Hospital of Lanzhou University, China

2 Department of Obstetrics and Gynecology, Key Laboratory for Gynecologic Oncology Gansu Province, The First Hospital of Lanzhou University, China

3 University of Maryland, USA

4 Independent Scholar

5 Cleveland Clinic, Lerner Research Institute, USA

6 Kent State University, USA

*Address all correspondence to: huangz@ccf.org and ylu13@kent.edu

† These authors contributed equally to this work.

References

[1] Wang TC. Yamada's Textbook of Gastroenterology. Hoboken, NJ: Wiley; 2022 p. 1 online resource

[2] Sylla P, Kaiser AM, Popowich D. The SAGES Manual of Colorectal Surgery. Cham: Springer; 2020 p. 1 online resource

[3] Tersigni R, Prantera C. Crohn's Disease: A Multidisciplinary Approach. Dordrecht: Springer; 2010 xviii, p. 303

[4] Buratovich MA. Principles of Microbiology. Principles of Science. Amenia, NY, USA: Salem Press, a division of EBSCO Information Services; 2022 xxix, 697 pages

[5] Guandalini S, Dhawan A. Textbook of Pediatric Gastroenterology, Hepatology and Nutrition: A Comprehensive Guide to Practice. Cham: Springer; 2022 p. 1 online resource

[6] Shiotani A. Gastric cancer: With Special Focus on Studies from Japan. Singapore: Springer; 2019 p. viii, 201 pages

[7] Kamiya S, Backert S. *Helicobacter pylori* in Human Diseases, in Advances in Microbiology, Infectious Diseases and Public Health. Cham, Switzerland: Springer; 2019 p. xix, 284 pages

[8] Chichlowski M, Hale LP. Effects of Helicobacter infection on research: The case for eradication of Helicobacter from rodent research colonies. Comparative Medicine. 2009;**59**(1):10-17

[9] Yu Y et al. *Helicobacter pylori* infection and inflammatory bowel disease: A crosstalk between upper and lower digestive tract. Cell Death & Disease. 2018;**9**(10):961

[10] Wu XW et al. *Helicobacter pylori* infection and inflammatory bowel disease in Asians: A meta-analysis. World Journal of Gastroenterology. 2015;**21**(15):4750-4756

[11] Papamichael K, Konstantopoulos P, Mantzaris GJ. *Helicobacter pylori* infection and inflammatory bowel disease: Is there a link? World Journal of Gastroenterology. 2014;**20**(21):6374-6385

[12] Sun J. Inflammation, Infection, and Microbiome in Cancers: Evidence, Mechanisms, and Implications, in Physiology in Health and Disease. Cham, Switzerland: Springer; 2021 p. xii, 509 pages

[13] Kanoun O, Derbel N. Advanced Sensors for Biomedical Applications, in Smart Sensors, Measurement and Instrumentation. Cham: Springer; 2021 p. 1 online resource

[14] Nordenfelt P, Otto MW. Bacterial Pathogenesis: Methods and Protocols, in Springer Protocols. New York: Humana Press: Springer; 2017 p. xi, 357 pages

[15] Gracia-sancho J, Salvadó MJ. Gastrointestinal Tissue: Oxidative Stress and Dietary Antioxidants. London: Academic Press; 2017 xvii, 376 pages

[16] Suzuki H, Warren JR, Marshall BJ. *Helicobacter pylori*. Japan: Springer; 2016 p. x, 267 pages

[17] Lanas A. NSAIDs and Aspirin: Recent Advances and Implications for Clinical Management. Switzerland: Springer; 2016 p. 1 online resource

[18] Wang WL, Xu XJ. Correlation between Helicobacter pylori infection and Crohn's disease: A meta-analysis.

European Review for Medical and Pharmacological Sciences. 2019;**23**(23):10509-10516

[19] Rokkas T et al. The association between *Helicobacter pylori* infection and inflammatory bowel disease based on meta-analysis. United European Gastroenterology Journal. 2015;**3**(6):539-550

[20] Jones K. Cancer sourcebook: Basic consumer health information about major forms and stages of cancer, featuring facts about head and neck cancers, lung cancers, gastrointestinal cancers, genitourinary cancers, lymphomas, blood cell cancers, endocrine cancers, skin cancers, bone cancers, metastatic cancers, and more; along with facts about cancer treatments, cancer risks and prevention. In: Health Reference Series. Detroit, MI, USA: Omnigraphics; p. 2015 77 entries

[21] Yue M et al. Is *Helicobacter pylori* infection associated with celiac disease? A Meta-analysis. The Turkish Journal of Gastroenterology. 2022;**33**(3):205-212

[22] Luther J et al. Association between *Helicobacter pylori* infection and inflammatory bowel disease: A meta-analysis and systematic review of the literature. Inflammatory Bowel Diseases. 2010;**16**(6):1077-1084

[23] Wang WL, Xu XJ. Correlation between *Helicobacter pylori* infection and Crohn's disease: A meta-analysis. European Review for Medical and Pharmacological Sciences. Dec 2019;**23**(23):10509-10516. DOI: 10.26355/eurrev_201912_19691. PMID: 31841206

[24] Shirzad-Aski H et al. Association between *Helicobacter pylori* colonization and inflammatory bowel disease: A systematic review and Meta-analysis. Journal of Clinical Gastroenterology. 2021;**55**(5):380-392

[25] Castano-Rodriguez N et al. Dual role of Helicobacter and Campylobacter species in IBD: A systematic review and meta-analysis. Gut. 2017;**66**(2):235-249

[26] Ding ZH et al. The prevalence of *Helicobacter pylori* infection in inflammatory bowel disease in China: A case-control study. PLoS One. 2021;**16**(3):e0248427

[27] Chun HJ et al. Small Intestine Disease: A Comprehensive Guide to Diagnosis and Management. Singapore: Springer; 2022. p. 1 online resource

[28] Hohenberger W, Parker M. Lower Gastrointestinal Tract Surgery. Vol. 2, Open Procedures, in Springer Surgery Atlas Series. Cham: Springer; 2021 p. xvii, 614 pages

[29] Hyman N, Fleshner P, Strong S. Mastery of IBD Surgery. Cham: Springer; 2019 p. xi, 409 pages, color illustrations

[30] Kohlstadt I. Food and Nutrients in Disease Management. Boca Raton: CRC Press; 2009 xxii, 717 pages

[31] Wyllie R, Hyams JS, Kay M. Pediatric Gastrointestinal and Liver Disease. Sixth edition ed. Philadelphia, PA: Elsevier; 2021 xx, 1091 pages

[32] Zhong Y et al. The relationship between *Helicobacter pylori* and inflammatory bowel disease. Archives of Iranian Medicine. 2021;**24**(4):317-325

[33] Bartels LE et al. Diagnosis of *Helicobacter pylori* infection is associated with lower prevalence and subsequent incidence of Crohn's disease. Journal of Crohn's & Colitis. 2016;**10**(4):443-448

[34] Engstrand L, Graham DY. Microbiome and gastric Cancer. Digestive Diseases and Sciences. 2020;**65**(3):865-873

[35] Bartels LE, Dahlerup JF. Association of *Helicobacter pylori* and Crohn's disease incidence: An inversion reaction? Digestive Diseases and Sciences. 2017;**62**(9):2217-2219

[36] Xiang Z et al. *Helicobacter pylori* and Crohn's disease: A retrospective single-center study from China. World Journal of Gastroenterology. 2013;**19**(28):4576-4581

[37] Roka K et al. The prevalence of *Helicobacter pylori* gastritis in newly diagnosed children with inflammatory bowel disease. Helicobacter. 2014;**19**(5):400-405

[38] Lender N et al. Review article: Associations between *Helicobacter pylori* and obesity--an ecological study. Alimentary Pharmacology & Therapeutics. 2014;**40**(1):24-31

[39] Toscano EP et al. Epidemiological and clinical-pathological aspects of *Helicobacter pylori* infection in Brazilian children and adults. Gastroenterology Research and Practice. 2018;**2018**:8454125

[40] Shah A et al. Is there a link between *H. pylori* and the epidemiology of Crohn's disease? Digestive Diseases and Sciences. 2017;**62**(9):2472-2480

[41] Ananthakrishnan AN. Epidemiology and risk factors for IBD. Nature Reviews. Gastroenterology & Hepatology. 2015;**12**(4):205-217

[42] Singh S et al. Epidemiology, risk factors and management of cardiovascular diseases in IBD. Nature Reviews. Gastroenterology & Hepatology. 2015;**12**(1):26-35

[43] Luther J et al. *Helicobacter pylori* DNA decreases pro-inflammatory cytokine production by dendritic cells and attenuates dextran sodium sulphate-induced colitis. Gut. 2011;**60**(11):1479-1486

[44] Owyang SY et al. *Helicobacter pylori* DNA's anti-inflammatory effect on experimental colitis. Gut Microbes. 2012;**3**(2):168-171

[45] Kim JM et al. *Helicobacter pylori* vacuolating cytotoxin induces apoptosis via activation of endoplasmic reticulum stress in dendritic cells. Journal of Gastroenterology and Hepatology. 2015;**30**(1):99-108

[46] Dixon BREA, Hossain R, Patel RV, Algood HMS. Th17 cells in *Helicobacter pylori* infection: A dichotomy of help and harm. Infection and Immunity. 18 Oct 2019;**87**(11):e00363-19. DOI: 10.1128/IAI.00363-19. PMID: 31427446; PMCID: PMC6803329

[47] Bhuiyan TR et al. Th1 and Th17 responses to *Helicobacter pylori* in Bangladeshi infants, children and adults. PLoS One. 2014;**9**(4):e93943

[48] Ansari S, Yamaoka Y. Animal models and *Helicobacter pylori* infection. Journal of Clinical Medicine. 31 May 2022;**11**(11):3141. DOI: 10.3390/jcm11113141. PMID: 35683528; PMCID: PMC9181647

[49] Vital JS, Tanoeiro L, Lopes-Oliveira R, Vale FF. Biomarker characterization and prediction of virulence and antibiotic resistance from *Helicobacter pylori* next generation sequencing data. Biomolecules. 11 May 2022;**12**(5):691. DOI: 10.3390/biom12050691. PMID: 35625618; PMCID: PMC9138241

[50] Suzuki R et al. Genome-wide mutation analysis of Helicobacter pylori after inoculation to Mongolian gerbils. Gut Pathog. 2019;**11**:45

[51] Cooper TK et al. Research-relevant conditions and pathology of laboratory

mice, rats, gerbils, Guinea pigs, hamsters, naked mole rats, and rabbits. ILAR Journal. 2021;**62**(1-2):77-132

[52] Israel DA et al. *Helicobacter pylori* strain-specific differences in genetic content, identified by microarray, influence host inflammatory responses. The Journal of Clinical Investigation. 2001;**107**(5):611-620

[53] Oster P et al. The efficacy of Cancer immunotherapies is compromised by *Helicobacter pylori* infection. Frontiers in Immunology. 2022;**13**:899161

[54] Reyes VE, Peniche AG. *Helicobacter pylori* deregulates T and B cell Signaling to trigger immune evasion. Current Topics in Microbiology and Immunology. 2019;**421**:229-265

[55] Baj J, Forma A, Sitarz M, Portincasa P, Garruti G, Krasowska D, et al. *Helicobacter pylori* virulence factors-mechanisms of bacterial pathogenicity in the gastric microenvironment. Cells. 25 Dec 2020;**10**(1):27. DOI: 10.3390/cells10010027. PMID: 33375694; PMCID: PMC7824444

[56] Gravina AG et al. *Helicobacter pylori* and extragastric diseases: A review. World Journal of Gastroenterology. 2018;**24**(29):3204-3221

[57] Wang L et al. *Helicobacter pylori* and autoimmune diseases: Involving multiple systems. Frontiers in Immunology. 2022;**13**:833424

[58] Bravo D et al. *Helicobacter pylori* in human health and disease: Mechanisms for local gastric and systemic effects. World Journal of Gastroenterology. 2018;**24**(28):3071-3089

[59] Arnold IC, Muller A. *Helicobacter pylori*: Does gastritis prevent colitis? Inflamm Intest Dis. 2016;**1**(3):102-112

[60] Fujita Y et al. Ulcerative colitis relapse after *Helicobacter pylori* eradication in a 12-year-old boy with duodenal ulcer. BMC Gastroenterology. 2021;**21**(1):424

[61] Axelrad JE et al. The role of gastrointestinal pathogens in inflammatory bowel disease: A systematic review. Therapeutic Advances in Gastroenterology. 2021;**14**:17562848211004493

[62] Sultan S et al. Metabolic influences of gut microbiota Dysbiosis on inflammatory bowel disease. Frontiers in Physiology. 2021;**12**:715506

[63] Raoul P, Cintoni M, Palombaro M, Basso L, Rinninella E, Gasbarrini A, et al. Food additives, a key environmental factor in the development of IBD through gut Dysbiosis. Microorganisms. 13 Jan 2022;**10**(1):167. DOI: 10.3390/microorganisms10010167. PMID: 35056616; PMCID: PMC8780106

[64] Zhang L et al. Bacterial species associated with human inflammatory bowel disease and their pathogenic mechanisms. Frontiers in Microbiology. 2022;**13**:801892

[65] Dann SM et al. Giardia infection of the small intestine induces chronic colitis in genetically susceptible hosts. Journal of Immunology. 2018;**201**(2):548-559

[66] Van Der Kraak LA et al. Genetic and commensal induction of IL-18 drive intestinal epithelial MHCII via IFNgamma. Mucosal Immunology. 2021;**14**(5):1100-1112

[67] Choi MS et al. *Helicobacter pylori*-derived outer membrane vesicles stimulate interleukin 8 secretion through nuclear factor kappa B activation. The Korean Journal of Internal Medicine. 2021;**36**(4):854-867

[68] Uotani T et al. Changes of tight junction and interleukin-8 expression

using a human gastroid monolayer model of *Helicobacter pylori* infection. Helicobacter. 2019;**24**(3):e12583

[69] Alexander SM et al. *Helicobacter pylori* in human stomach: The inconsistencies in clinical outcomes and the probable causes. Frontiers in Microbiology. 2021;**12**:713955

[70] Mladenova I. Clinical relevance of *Helicobacter pylori* infection. Journal of Clinical Medicine. 2021;**10**:3473. DOI: 10.3390/jcm10163473

[71] Taylor JM et al. Effects of a Th1-versus a Th2-biased immune response in protection against *Helicobacter pylori* challenge in mice. Microbial Pathogenesis. 2008;**44**(1):20-27

[72] Lindenberg M et al. Clarithromycin impairs tissue-resident memory and Th17 responses to macrolide-resistant *Streptococcus pneumoniae* infections. Journal of Molecular Medicine (Berlin, Germany). 2021;**99**(6):817-829

[73] Liu J et al. Erythromycin suppresses the cigarette smoke extract-exposed dendritic cell-mediated polarization of CD4(+) T cells into Th17 cells. Journal of Immunology Research. 2020;**2020**:1387952

[74] Takemori N et al. Possible mechanisms of action of clarithromycin and its clinical application as a repurposing drug for treating multiple myeloma. Ecancermedicalscience. 2020;**14**:1088

[75] Liu W et al. Mechanism of TH2/TH17-predominant and neutrophilic TH2/TH17-low subtypes of asthma. The Journal of Allergy and Clinical Immunology. 2017;**139**(5):1548-1558 e4

[76] Kim JJE et al. Efficacy of clarithromycin depends on the bacterial density in clarithromycin-Heteroresistant *Helicobacter pylori* infections: An In situ detected susceptibility and quantitative morphometry-based retrospective study. Pathology Oncology Research. 2021;**27**:1609863

[77] Mishima K et al. Lansoprazole upregulates Polyubiquitination of the TNF receptor-associated factor 6 and facilitates Runx2-mediated Osteoblastogenesis. eBioMedicine. 2015;**2**(12):2046-2061

Chapter 7

The Influence of *Helicobacter pylori* Infection Treatment on Psoriasis Severity

Sampson Weytey

Abstract

Helicobacter pylori infection is a condition caused by the gram-negative bacterium *H. pylori* affecting the mucous lining of the antrum portion of the stomach. At least 50% of the global population fall victim to this condition with Africans proven to have the highest prevalence rate of 70%, followed by South America and Western Asia with 69.4 and 66.6% respectively. In Africa, Nigeria is said to have the highest prevalence rate of *H. pylori* infection recording 87.7 to 89.7%. *H. pylori* infection is known to inflict a wide range of gastric complications including Peptic ulcer disease among others, and extra gastric complications such as Neurological diseases, as well as Dermatological diseases. Psoriasis, an autoimmune chronic inflammatory disease of the skin, affecting more than 100 million individuals globally, is one of the dermatological complications of *H. pylori* infection. It has been noted that *H. pylori* seem to play a major role in the development of psoriasis. Therefore, this chapter seeks to provide readers with the connection between *H. pylori* infection and Psoriasis as well as the influence the treatment of *H. pylori* infection has on Psoriasis severity.

Keywords: *Helicobacter pylori*, infection, antrum, psoriasis, dermatological, autoimmune, chronic, inflammatory, disease

1. Introduction

1.1 *Helicobacter pylori*

Helicobacter pylori (*H. pylori*) infection has over the years posed a global health burden significance, having a worldwide prevalence of 4.4 billion infected individuals approximately [1]. It has persisted for multiple decades among individuals at different part of the world, having a prevalence rate of 50% in the western world and an 80% prevalence rate among the population living in developing countries [2, 3]. A systematic review was carried out and it revealed that Africa, South America, and Western Asia had *H. pylori* infection prevalence rates of 70.1, 69.4, and 66.6%, respectively [4]. Epidemiological studies have projected Nigeria and South Africa to be the African nations experiencing high prevalence rates of 91 and 87% respectively when it comes to *H. pylori* infection, and 23% among Canadian adults in the Western world [5]. A systematic study conducted by Awuku et al. supported the fact that the adult population in developing countries has a higher prevalence rate of *H. pylori* infection as compared to children under 5 years with 90 and 50% respectively, whereas in developed countries like the USA has a higher prevalence rate of 10% among the adolescent individuals and 5% among children under 5 years of age [6]. A study conducted in Uganda by Aitala et al. shows that *H. pylori* infection among children varies with increasing ages ranging from 1 to 5 years, 6 to 10, and 11 to 15 with 16.2, 27.2, and 36.71% as their respective prevalence rate [7].

In 1982, two Australian researchers, Barry Marshall and Robin Warren conduct a study that included biopsies from 100 patients, and observed the presence of small, curved bacteria which will later be called *Helicobacter pylori*, in the lower stomachs in nearly all patients with gastric inflammation, duodenal ulcers, and stomach ulcers [8]. After this vital effort in the field of gastroenterology gained global recognition by the National Institutes of Health Consensus Development Conference in 1994, Food and Drug Administration (FDA) in 1996, and Centers for Disease Control and Prevention (CDC) in 1997, the Nobel Prize Foundation awarded Marshall and Warren a Nobel Prize in physiology and medicine later in the year 2005 [1, 8]. Recent studies have identified *H. pylori* to play a major role in the development of diseases such as gastritis and mucosa-associated lymphoid tissue (MALT)lymphoma, as well as peptic ulcer and gastric cancer [1].

Helicobacter pylori infection is caused by the gram-negative micro bacterium *Helicobacter pylori* (*H. pylori*), which is helicoidal, unipolar, and multiflagellate in nature having the tendency to cause gastritis, peptic ulcer disease (PUD) as well as gastric cancer by inhabiting the gastric mucosa of its victim [9]. It has an average length that ranges from 2.5 to 5.0 μm and width from 0.5 to 1.0 μm [10]. H. pylorus is a slow-growing microbe that can be cultured both on none selective agar media such as blood or chocolate agar and on selective agar media such as Skirrow's media incubated at 35 to 37°C in a 5% oxygen atmosphere for 3 to 7 days [11]. This microorganism possesses 2 to 7 unipolar sheathed flagella rising from a smooth and rounded outer membrane which enhances its mobility through viscous solutions [12]. Under hostile conditions like stressed, old, or mal-nutritious and prolonged air exposure cultures, the microbe can become dormant enabling its long-term adaptation and survival in less favorable environment outside of the host organism [13]. Electron microscopic studies have identified that *Helicobacter pylori* can exist in spiral forms that are viable, can be cultured, virulent, and can infect experimental animals to cause inflammation [14]. The second form is the coccoid form, where the microbe is viable, but cannot be cultured and is less virulent to colonize or cause inflammation in experimental animals [14]. The final form is degenerative, and this form cannot be cultured and is considered as the death form of *H. pylori* [14].

Numerous epidemiological studies have demonstrated that eating contaminated foods, living in crowded areas, having a low socioeconomic status, and practicing poor personal and environmental hygiene are the main risk factors for contracting *H. pylori* infection, particularly in developing nations [15, 16]. Additionally, it has been established that swimming in rivers, streams, or pools increases one's risk of *H. pylori* infection by three times as compared to non-swimmers [14]. The *H. pylori* bacteria can be found in close proximity to human environments in animals including cows, cats, dogs, and sheep, placing nearby people at risk of contracting the infection [17].

Few works of literature have been provided on the main route of infection, however, in both developing and developed nations, *H. pylori* infection occurs throughout infancy or adolescence and can spread through oral-oral or fecal-oral, person-to-person, as well as through zoonotic transmission [17–19]. *H. pylori* infection routes confined to the person–person transmission can be conceivable through direct contact with the saliva, vomit, or feces of the infected person, as well as from nursing mothers, family members, or caretakers even to babies at the early stages of life [7, 20]. Genetic susceptibility in the development of *H. pylori* infections is also possible in according to scientific studies [21]. Vertical and horizontal transmission are the two primary divisions of person-to-person transmission [22]. The spread of infection among members of the same family is the vertical mode of transmission, whereas the horizontal form of transmission includes contamination among individuals outside the family [22].

Gastric adenocarcinoma and mucosa-associated lymphoid tissue (MALT) lymphoma have been associated with *Helicobacter pylori*, a causative agent of gastritis and peptic ulcers [23]. *H. pylori*'s capacity to produce this range of illnesses is influenced by host, bacterial, and environmental variables [15, 24]. Urease, flagella, adhesins, δ-glutamyltranspeptidase, lipopolysaccharide, and vacuolating, cytotoxin are some of the bacterial components required for *H. pylori* to colonize the stomach mucosa, remain for decades, and cause a severe inflammatory response that damages host cells [15]. Non-steroidal anti-inflammatory medicines (NSAID), alcohol, and smoking are examples of environmental factors, and host factors like gene polymorphism and immune response can also play a role [24]. Despite the stomach's unfavorable environment, *H. pylori* can use it as its principal site of colonization and survive there for years [1]. The four main steps necessary for *H. pylori* colonization and pathogenesis are as follows: (1) surviving in the acidic environment of the stomach; (2) moving toward epithelium cells through flagella-mediated motility; (3) attaching to host receptors by adhesins; and (4) inflicting tissue damage by releasing toxins [25]. At each crucial stage, *H. pylori* engages in a particular strategic activity to promote effective colonization, persistent infection, and disease pathogenesis [24]. In order to evade the stomach's acidic environment and spread a chronic infection, the pathogen first enters the host stomach lumen and then localizes to the antrum and corpus for adaption before it neutralizes the stomach's hostile acidic environment with its urease activity [26, 27]. Following effective colonization and sustained infection, *H. pylori* must first migrate toward the host gastric epithelial cells using flagella-mediated motility. Next, specific interactions between bacterial adhesins and host cell receptors ensue [27]. At last, cytotoxin-associated gene A (CagA) and vacuolating cytotoxin A (VacA), among others, are released by *H. pylori* to cause damage to the host's tissues [27]. Additionally, the gastric epithelial layer, which functions as the main point of contact between *H. pylori* and the host, secretes chemokines that stimulate neutrophils and start innate immunity, which in turn causes clinical illnesses like gastritis and peptic ulcer to develop [27].

Studies have shown that most *Helicobacter pylori* infections are asymptomatic, with about 30–35% of patients showing no symptoms, which is frequently seen in young people [28]. According to one school of thought, the host's genetics, the properties of the bacteria, and the environment can all interact to cause a variety of clinical symptoms in the affected person [21]. Research among students found that nausea (25.5%), gastrointestinal discomfort (24.5%), and heartburn (20.2%) were the most common symptoms linked to *H. pylori* infections, followed by vomiting (12.8%), appetite loss (5.3%), and dyspepsia (3.2%) [29]. Some signs and symptoms commonly associated with *H. pylori* infection include fatigue, weakness, digestive bleeding, gastric reflux, weight loss, low appetite, bloating in the belly, dark stools, frequent burping, nausea, vomiting, gnawing or searing stomach pain [30, 31]. Although it can happen at other times, abdominal pain typically manifests itself in the early morning hours, between meals, and when the stomach is empty [32]. Late eradication of the *H. pylori* infection can be accompanied by both gastric and extra-gastric complications [33, 34]. *Helicobacter pylori* infection is the primary cause of gastric complications such as chronic gastritis, gastric ulcer, duodenal ulcer, gastric adenocarcinoma and gastric mucosa-associated lymphoid tissue (MALT) lymphoma [35], and associated extra-gastric complications, including Allergic Diseases, Metabolic Diseases, Neurological Diseases, Inflammatory Bowel Diseases, Esophageal Diseases, Dermatologic Diseases, Ophthalmic Diseases, Hematological Diseases [36, 37].

Many gastroduodenal illnesses can be effectively treated and eradicated if *H. pylori* infection is early and correctly diagnosed [38]. There are both invasive and non-invasive diagnostic methods for the identification of *H. pylori*, and each test has benefits and drawbacks depending on the clinical situation [18, 38]. Although there is no single technique that can be used as the gold standard in clinical practice, numerous have been established and are necessary to get more accurate outcomes [38]. Endoscopic biopsy samples are used for invasive procedures, such as histology, culture, fast urease test, and molecular techniques [18, 39]. The real-time diagnosis of *H. pylori* during endoscopy is also made possible by advancements in endoscopic technology [38]. The most used non-invasive diagnostic methods are the urea breathing test and stool antigen test, whereas serology is beneficial for screening and epidemiological research [39]. Other than gastric mucosa, variable specimens have been studied using molecular approaches [38]. In addition to the *H. pylori* infection test, other tests are used to screen for precancerous lesions, gastric cancer, and *H. pylori* virulence factors and antibiotic sensitivity [38, 39]. In order to lower the prevalence of antibiotic resistance, the American College of Gastroenterology (ACG) advises testing in patients with symptoms of dyspepsia, active peptic ulcer disease, and gastric mucosa-associated lymphoid tissue (MALT) lymphoma [40, 41].

Following endoscopic resection for an *H. pylori*-positive gastric adenoma [42], *H. pylori* eradication can be advised, and the chosen treatment plan should have an eradication rate of at least 90% [43, 44], to prevent local recurrence and to improve dyspeptic symptoms over the long term in patients with functional dyspepsia [45, 46]. There are other *H. pylori* treatment plans, including triple therapy, sequential therapy (the patient receives one treatment, then another), quadruple therapy, and triple therapy based on levofloxacin [45]. Studies have demonstrated that the eradication regimen is an effective management in reducing *H. pylori* infection linked with gastric cancer and extra-gastric complications [43]. Single and dual medication regimens have unacceptably poor cure rates and are not advised, but triple and quadruple therapies have shown eradication rates approaching 90% or higher [1, 43]. The goal of treating an *H. pylori* infection is to eradicate the *H. pylori* microbe, heal an ulcer that may be present in the duodenum or stomach, and avoid a recurrence of the infection, which may occur after 7 to 14 days of treatment [42]. In the treatment of the infection, antisecretory agents are used in combination with antimicrobial agents to achieve the bactericidal effect [1].

The bacterium can be eliminated with antibiotics such as Amoxicillin, Clarithromycin, Metronidazole, Tetracycline, or Tinidazole [47]. By preventing the stomach from producing gastric acid, Dexlansoprazole, Esomeprazole, Lansoprazole, or Omeprazole can reduce the amount of gastric acid secreted [47]. Common histamine H2-receptor antagonists (H2 blockers) like Cimetidine, Famotidine, Nizatidine, and Ranitidine are used to prevent histamine from mediating the production of gastric acid, which is necessary to erode the lining of the stomach [47]. Surgery is not a viable option for those with *H. pylori* infection and should only be suggested for those who are experiencing serious problems, such as malignancies [42]. Amoxicillin, Clarithromycin, and Proton-pump inhibitor (PPI) for a period of 14 days have been selected as the first-line eradication management for routine triple therapy [21, 42]. It has been shown that PPI, Metronidazole, Amoxicillin, and Clarithromycin have an eradication efficiency rate of 84.3% [15]. Even after treatment, patients must undergo another test to ensure that the *Helicobacter pylori* infection has been completely eliminated [21]. Sequential therapy has been shown to achieve positive outcomes with an efficiency rate greater than 90% in the eradication therapy technique [48]. The length of the eradication therapy is also crucial, and studies and recommendations from the European and American medical communities suggest that a consecutive 14-day course of treatment is the most effective among durations of 7, 10, or 14 days [48].

It is crucial that clinicians inform patients about the consequences of noncompliance because *H. pylori* antibiotic resistance, which is rising in most of the world, is a significant factor in treatment failure [44]. This resistance is brought on by decreased adherence to clinical regimens and nutrition therapies [43]. It has been demonstrated that a compliance rate of less than 80% reduces treatment effectiveness [44]. A medication susceptibility test should be performed before taking therapy in order to determine the appropriate regimen required for precise management [49]. Due to the rising abuse and overuse of antibiotics for the treatment of various infections in the majority of developing countries, *H. pylori* infection has a higher prevalence rate of antibiotic resistance than other bacteria [15]. Antibiotic resistance in young people is a result of some contributing variables, such as the failure to respond to therapy and inadequate gastric suppressants [42]. The World Health Organization (WHO) highlighted *H. pylori* resistance in 2017 as a significant factor in the treatment of *H. pylori* and as a prevalent source of community-acquired infection [15]. Since first-line therapy has been found to have a failure rate of roughly 20%, it has been suggested that second-line therapy be added to eliminate *H. pylori* [49].

1.2 Psoriasis

Psoriasis is a chronic, immune-mediated inflammatory skin disease, characterize by red, scaly plaques occurring most commonly on the elbows, knees, scalp, and lower back, as well as any part of the skin surface [50]. The condition greatly affects people's quality of life to the extent that it could be life-ruining and stigmatizing [50, 51]. Psoriasis is now considered a systemic disease and is associated with psychological, metabolic, arthritic, and cardiovascular comorbidities [50, 52], which have been proven by epidemiological studies to reduce the lifespan of affected individuals [50]. In addition to the psychological and social burden related to psoriasis, the cost to patients and healthcare systems is high [50, 53]. Psoriasis can occur at any age, although most patients present with the condition before 35 years old [50].

Psoriasis has probably been as old as modern man and has also been reported in non-human primates, but was recognized as a disease in the nineteenth century [51]. The root word of psoriasis was derived from the Greek word 'Psora', referred to as itch [51]. For centuries, patients with psoriasis suffered the same cruel fate as lepers because there was random grouping together of all inflammatory skin diseases which brought about the stigmatization of patients with psoriasis until it was separated from leprosy and its significant signs and types were also identified [51]. Essential signs were discovered by great physicians over the years such as the recognition of the Auspitz sign, Köbner's phenomenon, Munro's abscesses, generalized pustular psoriasis, and the Woronoff ring have provided important diagnostic tools which allowed physicians to be more confident in diagnosing psoriasis these days [51]. Today in the twenty first century, psoriasis is no longer regarded simply as a skin condition, but as a chronic autoimmune disease, characterized by systemic inflammation which affects not just the skin, but also joints and other bodily systems [51].

Psoriasis is a common chronic inflammatory disease with a prevalence rate of 0.33–0.6% in different races and affects approximately 125 million people worldwide [53]. Based on the 2020 US census data, there were an estimated 7.55 million US adults with psoriasis [54]. White individuals have been identified to have the prevalence rate of 3.6%, followed by other racial/ethnic groups (non-Hispanic, including multiracial) at 3.1%, Asian individuals at 2.5%, Hispanic individuals (including Mexican American and other Hispanic individuals) at 1.9%, and Black individuals at 1.5% [54]. Systematic reviews have revealed that psoriasis prevalence in children in Italy is approximately 2.1% and that the rates among adults vary from 0.4% in Asian countries to 8.5% in Norway [50, 54]. Higher prevalence rates have been reported at higher latitudes and in white people compared to other ethnic groups [50]. Adults were more likely than children to develop psoriasis [50]. From 0.02% (95% confidence interval 0.01 to 0.04%) in east Asia to 0.22% (0.06 to 0.81%) in Australasia and 0.21% (0.11 to 0.41%) in western Europe, psoriasis prevalence in children varies [50, 54]. From 0.14% (0.05 to 0.40%) in east Asia to 1.99% (0.64 to 6.60%) in Australasia, the disease affected adults in different ways [50]. Western Europe (1.92, 1.07 to 3.46%), central Europe (1.83, 0.62 to 5.32%), high-income North America (1.50, 0.63 to 3.60%), and high-income southern Latin America (1.10, 0.36 to 2.96%) were other locations with an occurrence rate of the disease above 1% [50, 53]. The scalp (43.0%; 1726/4016) was the area of the body most commonly afflicted by psoriasis that was difficult to cure, followed by the face (29.9%; 1200/4016), nails (24.5%; 982/4016), soles (15.6%; 628/4016), genitals (14.1%; 568/4016), and palms (13.7%; 551/4016), in that order [53]. Sixty-two percent (2602/4016), 42% (1702/4016), and 29% (878/4016) of all patients, respectively, had involvement in one or more, two or more, or three or more hard-to-treat areas [53].

There are several risk factors that can contribute to the development of psoriasis [55]. Today, it has been recognized that psoriasis results from a complex interaction between immunological, genetic, cellular, and environmental factors [51, 52, 55]. Since many people with psoriasis have a family history of the condition, researchers have identified a few genes that may be involved in its onset [52]. These genes all have an impact on how well the immune system works. The risk of having psoriasis may be increased by a number of extrinsic causes, like smoking, obesity, stress, cold temperatures, skin injuries, and certain races may also predispose a person to certain infections, including streptococcal and HIV infections, as well as some medications for treating heart disease, malaria, or mental health issues [55].

The dermatologic manifestations of psoriasis can be classified into different groups depending on their characteristics [56]. Nail psoriasis is the type that affects the fingernails and toenails, causing pitting, abnormal nail growth, and discoloration [56]. Young people and children are most commonly affected by Guttate psoriasis, which is characterized by small, drop-shaped patches of scaling on the trunk, arms, or legs and is typically brought on by a bacterial infection like strep throat [52]. Smooth patches of inflammatory skin that get worse with friction and perspiration are the main symptoms of inverse psoriasis, which primarily affects the skin folds of the groin, buttocks, and breasts [55]. This kind of psoriasis may be brought on by fungi [52]. A rare form of psoriasis called Pustular psoriasis can affect tiny portions of the palms or soles or form large patches with distinct pus-filled blisters [56]. The least frequent type of psoriasis, Erythrodermic psoriasis can cover the entire body with a peeling rash that can itch or burn violently and is typically short-term (acute) or long-term (chronic) [55]. The most prevalent form of psoriasis is Plaque psoriasis [56], which results in scale-covered, dry, elevated skin patches (plaques) [52]. They might be few or numerous and typically show up on the scalp, lower back, elbows, and knees [56]. The color of the patches varies depending on the skin tone, and on dark or Black skin, in particular, the afflicted skin may recover with transitory color changes (post-inflammatory hyperpigmentation) [56]. Joints are impacted by Psoriatic arthritis, which is typically a severe case of psoriasis [55]. The final one is Sebo-psoriasis, a kind of psoriasis that crosses with seborrheic dermatitis and often manifests on the face and scalp as red bumps and plaques with a greasy yellow scale [52].

The hallmark of psoriasis is sustained inflammation that leads to uncontrolled keratinocyte proliferation and dysfunctional differentiation [52]. The histology of the psoriatic plaque shows epidermal hyperplasia of about 10 times the usual [51], and the inflammatory infiltrates are composed of dermal dendritic cells, macrophages, T cells, and neutrophils [52]. This epidermal hyperplasia process results in the thickening, crusting and scaling of the skin [51]. Neovascularization is also a prominent feature [52]. The inflammatory pathways active in plaque psoriasis and the rest of the clinical variants overlap but also display discrete differences that account for the different phenotypes and treatment outcomes [52]. The process in psoriatic patients can occur in only 2 days [52]. It soon became clear that the high turnover of epidermal cells was caused by a series of autoimmune reactions, in which a portion of the body's immune system overreacts and targets healthy tissues [51, 52]. Following the production of certain inflammatory chemicals called cytokines, the resultant inflammation causes reddish, thickened, dry, and scaly skin as characteristics of psoriasis [51, 52, 56]. It has also been identified that psoriatic disease blocks the action of a specific type of immune cell called a T-cell, or they block inflammatory proteins (cytokines) such as tumor necrosis factor-alpha (TNF-alpha), and interleukins (17A, 12, and 23) which play an essential role in the development of the skin and joint manifestations of psoriasis [51].

The signs and symptoms of psoriasis can vary depending on the type of psoriasis present in the individual [55]. The following are the top five psoriasis signs and symptoms: Rashes or red, inflammatory skin patches that are frequently covered in loose, silver-colored scales [55]. In more severe cases, the plaques will spread and converge, covering substantial amounts [52, 55]. Scratching itchy, irritated skin can cause small patches of the skin to split or bleed [55]. Psoriasis can also be associated with psoriatic arthritis, which causes achy, swollen joints, usually common in approximately 10–30% of people with psoriasis [53–55].

People with psoriasis may also be more likely to get certain complications such as cancers, Crohn's disease, diabetes, metabolic syndrome, obesity, osteoporosis, uveitis (inflammation of the middle of the eye), liver disease, metabolic diseases, cardiovascular diseases, such as heart attacks, strokes, chronic kidney disease (CKD), gastrointestinal diseases, malignancy, mood disorders, infections and psoriatic arthritis (PsA), and mental health problems, such as low self-esteem, anxiety, depression as well as psoriatic arthritis, a chronic form of arthritis that causes pain, swelling, and stiffness of the joints and places where tendons and ligaments attach to bones (entheses) [55].

Psoriasis is primarily diagnosed through clinical means [56]. The most prevalent clinical form of psoriasis, which affects 80–90% of psoriasis sufferers, is chronic plaque psoriasis [56]. Erythematous plaques that are clearly defined, symmetrical, and covered in a silvery scale are the distinguishing features of classic plaque psoriasis [56].

In a physical examination, the skin is examined to identify lesions and note their distribution, size, form, and appearance [57]. During a physical exam, the psoriatic patient may be asked about his or her symptoms, medical and family history [57]. Also, a Skin Biopsy may be required to accurately diagnose the type of psoriasis [58].

Treatment of psoriasis is still based on controlling the symptoms [55]. Topical and systemic therapies as well as phototherapy are available in the treatment of psoriasis [51]. In practice, a combination of these methods is often used, and treatment is usually lifelong which is aimed at remission [52, 53]. Scientific research has proved that care for patients with psoriasis requires not only treating skin lesions, stopping skin cells from growing so quickly, removing scales and joint involvement, but it is also very important to identify and manage common comorbidity that already exists or may have developed, including cardiovascular and metabolic diseases as well as psychological conditions [51, 55]. Treatments may depend on how severe the psoriasis is and how responsive it has been to previous treatment and self-care measures [54]. Topical therapy may involve the use of Corticosteroids, Vitamin D analogs, Retinoids, Tazarotene, Calcineurin inhibitors, Salicylic acid, Coal tar, and Anthralin [50, 55]. Light therapy is a first-line treatment for moderate to severe psoriasis, either alone or in combination with medications [52]. It involves exposing the skin to controlled amounts of natural or artificial light [52]. The use of light therapy includes Sunlight, Goeckerman therapy, Ultraviolet B (UVB) broadband, Ultraviolet B (UVB) narrowband, Psoralen plus ultraviolet A (PUVA), and Excimer laser [52]. Oral or injected medications may include Steroids, Biologics, Methotrexate, and Cyclosporine [52].

2. *Helicobacter pylori* and psoriasis

2.1 Positive correlation

Onsun et al. studied the prevalence of *H. pylori* seropositivity in psoriasis patients, the link between PASI (Psoriasis Area and Severity Index) scores and *H. pylori* infection, and the effect of *H. pylori* infection on treatment response. To ascertain the prevalence of *H. pylori* seropositivity in psoriasis, the association between PASI scores and *H. pylori* infection, and the effect of *H. pylori* infection on the response to treatment, 300 patients with plaque-type psoriasis and 150 non-psoriatic healthy controls were studied. Both patients and controls had a stool antigen test for *H. pylori*. PASI scores were used to evaluate each patient's illness severity. From 184 *H. pyloric*-infected psoriatic patients, 50 were chosen at random. These 50 were divided into two groups, with the first group (n = 25) receiving acitretin monotherapy and the second group (n = 25) receiving *H. pyloric* treatment. Twenty-five (25) patients who only underwent *H. pyloric* treatment without receiving any systemic therapy were also contrasted with the two groups. The PASI scores of the patients were assessed and contrasted 8 weeks later. Psoriatic patients (n = 184) had a 61.3% prevalence of *H. pylori* infection, compared to 59.3% in controls (n = 89/150; P > 0.05). Patients who received both acitretin and treatment for *H. pylori* infection improved more quickly than those who received only acitretin (mean PASI score drop, 3.38 ± 1.99; P < 0.001 vs. 1.22 ± 0.77; P < 0.05). Patients who solely underwent *H. pylori* therapy showed significant improvement compared to controls (mean PASI score decreased from 2.85 to 1.25; P < 0.001). According to this research, *H. pylori* infections may contribute to the severity of psoriasis, and eliminating them will improve the effectiveness of psoriasis treatment [59].

A case–control study was conducted on 40 patients with psoriasis Vulgaris and 40 age-matched and sex-matched healthy individuals. The aim of the study was to clarify the role of *Helicobacter pylori* infection in psoriatic patients with palm and sole affection. This case–control study was conducted at the Dermatology, Andrology, and Sexually transmitted diseases and Medical Biochemistry Departments of the Faculty of Medicine, Menoufia University. Every patient underwent a thorough medical examination and history taking. Using an enzyme-linked immunosorbent test, the anti-*H. pylori* immunoglobulin G levels in the blood were determined. Statistics were used to compare anti-*H. pylori* immunoglobulin G serum levels to psoriasis area and severity index score. Patients with Psoriasis Vulgaris of either sex who had not previously received either systemic (3 months) or topical (2 weeks) treatment for their psoriasis met the inclusion criteria. Exclusion criteria included patients with other dermatological diseases except for psoriasis Vulgaris, patients with autoimmune diseases such as systemic lupus erythematosus, patients with inflammatory bowel diseases, patients with chronic diseases such as chronic renal failure, and patients having infectious conditions at the time of blood sampling such as bacterial infections [60].

In the PASI score, the body is divided into four sections: head (H), arms (A), trunk (T), and legs (L). Each of these areas is scored by itself, and then the four scores are combined into the final PASI score. In each of these areas, the percentage of the total surface area that was impacted was graded on a scale from 0 to 6, where grade 0 corresponds to 0% of the involved area, grade 1 to less than 10%, grade 2 to 10–29%, grade 3 to 30–49%, grade 4 to 50–69%, grade 5 to 70–89%, and grade 6 to 90–100% of the involved area. According to the findings, patients who did not exhibit palm and sole affection had a higher prevalence of *H. pylori* infection. However, 50% of palm-affected and sole-affected patients were positive for *H. pylori* infection ($P = 0.02$). Therefore, it was concluded that *H. pylori* may play a significant role in the development of palmoplantar psoriasis and may provide important clues to assist in the development of new therapeutic strategies for palmoplantar psoriatic patients through its eradication [60].

Fathy et al. conducted a study with the aim to evaluate the occurrence of *H. pylori* infection in chronic plaque-type psoriasis patients in order to determine a possible contribution to the pathogenesis of psoriasis. They compared 20 patients with chronic plaque-type psoriasis with 20 healthy, age- and sex-matched controls for *H. pylori* infection by using *H. pylori* IgG quantitative enzyme immunoassay (ELISA test). Patients under the age of 18, women who were expecting or nursing babies, and anyone who had taken antibiotics 40 days or histamine H2-receptor antagonists (H2 blockers) 14 days before sample withdrawal were all excluded from the study. Patients with peptic ulcer disease, gastrointestinal tract complaints, autoimmune or skin conditions, or those who had received therapy for psoriasis in the past were also disqualified. Every candidate conducted a background check, paying particular attention to their psoriasis history (onset, precipitating factors, course, and duration of the disease). Clinical examination revealed that the patients had persistent plaque-type psoriasis. The severity and breadth of psoriasis were assessed using the Psoriasis Area and Severity Index (PASI score). Greater values were associated with more severe psoriasis. In psoriatic patients, the mean (SD) prevalence of *H. pylori* IgG seropositivity was considerably higher than in controls (67.7 ± 32.5 vs. 33.9 ± 15.1; $P < 0.05$). These findings can support the hypothesis that *H. pylori* and psoriasis are related. For a definitive confirmation, large-scale investigations and additional research are needed for psoriatic patients who are *H. pylori* seropositive [61].

2.2 Negative correlation

A study conducted by Cinar et al. at Ankara Numune Education and Research Hospital Dermatology Department among 120 histopathologically diagnosed psoriasis patients and seropositive for *Helicobacter pylori*. The aim of the study was to evaluate the possible effect of *Helicobacter pylori* eradication on the psoriasis course. The *Helicobacter pylori* positivity was established using the carbon-14 urea breath test. The study also excluded patients under the age of 18 and those who had used any systemic medication within the previous 6 months or any topical medication other than emollients within the previous month. The psoriasis area severity index was used to assess the severity of the disease (PASI). At the commencement, at the conclusion of the eradication therapy (15th day), and at the 30th day, the patient's psoriasis area severity index (PASI) scores were computed. The difference in the mean PASI score between the two groups was compared. The study did not include anyone with a PASI score higher than 10. After the confirmation of H. pylori positivity, eighty (80) of the patients were given eradication therapy for H. pylori for fourteen (14) days which were clarithromycin (500 mg/twice daily), lansoprazole (30 mg/twice daily), and amoxicillin (1000 mg/twice daily). Forty psoriasis patients were chosen to be in the control group. The patients in the control group were not given any medication for H. pylori eradication. The mean age and sex distribution between the patient and control groups were similar. Prior to therapy, the body mass indices (BMI) of the patients were also determined to identify whether there would be a correlation between the BMI and *H. pylori* eradication response. The study's findings revealed a statistically significant decline in the treatment group's mean PASI score in percentage terms on both the 15th and 30th days. However, there was no discernible difference in the groups' PASI-50 or PASI-75 responses. The patients' responses to eradication therapy did not correlate with their body mass indices. So it was concluded that although there was a decrease in the mean PASI scores after eradication therapy, the number of patients who had a PASI-50 response was not significant, hence *H. pylori* eradication is not effective in healing psoriasis [62].

A case–control study was done on 61 patients with Psoriasis Vulgaris (cases) and 61 healthy individuals (controls) in Fatemiye Hospital (referral center for the treatment of skin diseases), Semnan, Iran. The aim of this study was to determine the relationship between *H. pylori* seropositivity and psoriasis. The Semnan University of Medical Sciences ethical commission in Iran gave its approval before the study could begin. The inclusion criteria were met by otherwise healthy people who had seen a dermatologist for cosmetic issues (control group) and patients with known Psoriasis Vulgaris (case group). Excluded from the study were patients having a history of gastrointestinal issues, those who had taken oral corticosteroids or b-blockers, or who had used topical or systemic treatment for 2 or 6 months, respectively. Prior to starting treatment, psoriatic patients had a clinical evaluation based on the PASI score and percentage of body surface area affected. To assess the severity of skin illness, the PASI was utilized. The effect of IgG against *H. pylori* was examined in all patients using an enzyme-linked immunosorbent assay (ELISA) kit (DRG Instruments, GmbH, Marburg, Germany) according to the manufacturer's protocol. Ten (16.4%) of the psoriatic patients and 8 (13%) of the control groups had an *H. pylori* seropositive test result; the average IgG serum level was 17.3 IU/ML in psoriatic patients and 16.1 IU/ML in the control group. The difference in serum levels between the two groups was not meaningful ($P = 0.302$). It was shown that neither the severity of psoriasis nor the serum level of IgG Anti-*H. pylori* were found to be significantly correlated with either the presence or absence of psoriasis. It was also suggested that more research be done to determine whether *H. pylori* infection is one of the factors causing or exacerbating psoriasis [63].

A nationwide population-based longitudinal cohort study was conducted with the aim to investigate the association between *H. pylori* infection and psoriasis. Between 2000 and 2013, the Longitudinal Health Insurance Research Database of the National Health Insurance Research Database in Taiwan yielded 41,539 patients with *H. pylori* infection and 83,078 matched controls for the study. To match the age, sex, comorbidities, and medical visits at a 1:2 ratio, propensity score analysis was employed. The adjusted hazard ratio of psoriasis was estimated using multiple Cox regression analysis. Additionally, stratified analysis and sensitivity testing were performed. Patients were excluded if they had ever been diagnosed with psoriasis before the index date, were diagnosed before 2000, or had undergone anti-*H. pylori* therapy before the index date or an appropriate propensity score-matched control could not be identified. Only patients who had been diagnosed with psoriasis at least three times at outpatient clinics, or were admitted at least once, were eligible for inclusion in the final analysis. Patients were disqualified if they had ever received a psoriasis diagnosis prior to the index date, had their condition diagnosed before the year 2000, or had had anti-*H. pylori* medication prior to the index date, or if a suitable propensity score-matched control could not be found. For inclusion in the final analysis, only patients who had received a psoriasis diagnosis at least three times at outpatient clinics or who had been hospitalized at least once were qualified [64].

In addition, it identified comorbidities related to *H. pylori* infection and psoriasis, namely systemic lupus erythematosus, ankylosing spondylitis, rheumatoid arthritis, Sjogren syndrome, hypertension, diabetes mellitus, hyperlipidemia, coronary artery disease, osteoporosis, cerebral vascular accident, asthma, chronic obstructive pulmonary disease and, chronic kidney disease, chronic liver diseases, chronic urticarial, tuberculosis, pneumonia, sepsis, and herpes zoster. Comorbidities were defined, using the relevant diagnostic codes, as at least one hospital admission or two outpatient visits of a given disease within 2 years before the index date. These comorbidities were considered covariates in the multivariate analysis [64].

Between the *H. pylori* and control cohorts, there were no appreciable differences in the incidence rates of psoriasis (4.58 vs. 4.20 per 100,000 person-months, crude relative risk: 1.092, 95% confidence interval: 0.917–1.302). In patients with *H. pylori* infection, there was no discernible difference in psoriasis risk after multivariate adjustment (adjusted hazard ratio: 1.081, 95% confidence interval: 0.907–1.288). Men, the elderly, people with diabetes, hyperlipidemia, chronic obstructive pulmonary disease, or tuberculosis all had a significantly greater risk of developing psoriasis. The stratified analysis also confirmed that *H. pylori* infection was not correlated with an increased risk of psoriasis based on follow-up duration, sex, and age. This retrospective population-based longitudinal cohort study, conducted in Taiwan, found no association between *H. pylori* infection and risk of psoriasis. Based on follow-up duration, sex, and age, the stratified analysis further indicated that *H. pylori* infection was not associated with a higher risk of psoriasis. No correlation between *H. pylori* infection and risk of psoriasis was discovered in this retrospective population-based longitudinal cohort investigation carried out in Taiwan [64].

3. Conclusion

Helicobacter pylori infection is a global health burden affecting not less than half the world's population for the past years. The gram-negative bacterium, *Helicobacter pylori* being its causative agent, also causes a broad spectrum of both gastric and extra gastric disorders among its victim. Dermatological diseases such as Psoriasis are known among the extra gastric disorders to be identified with *Helicobacter pylori*'s negative impact. Psoriasis is a chronic, immune-mediated inflammatory skin disease known to affect approximately 125 million individuals worldwide. Although some studies have presented the negative correlations between *H. pylori* and psoriasis, many more current studies have overridden the formal facts and have gone further to prove that *H. pylori* eradication has a positive influence on psoriasis severity.

Acknowledgements

Extending sincere gratitude to all authors and publishers of the books and articles used as references in this research work. Good wishes to all who will find this research work useful in their various field of study. Many appreciations and gratitude to the sponsors and funders of this research work. Thank you.

Author details

Sampson Weytey
School of Nursing, Valley View University, Accra, Ghana

*Address all correspondence to: sampsonweytey@gmail.com

References

[1] Oztenkin M, Yilmaz B, Agagunduz D, Capasso R. Overview of *Helicobacter* infection: Clinical feature, treatment, and nutritional aspects. Diseases. 2021;**9**(4):66. DOI: 10.3390/diseases 9040066

[2] Wu MC, Ma KS, Chen HH, Huanh JY, Wei JC. Relationship between *Helicobacter pylori* infection and psoriasis: A nationwide population-based longitudinal cohort study. Medicine. 2020;**99**(24):e20632. DOI: 10.1097/ MD.0000000000020632

[3] Magen E, Delgado JS. *Helicobacter pylori* and skin autoimmune disease. World Journal of Gastroenterology. 2014;**20**(6):1510-1516. DOI: 10:3748/wjg. v20.i6.1510

[4] Smith S, Fowora M, Pellicano R. Infections with *Helicobacter pylori* and challenges encountered in Africa. World Journal of Gastroenterology. 2019;**25**(25):3183-3195. DOI: 10.3748/wjg. v25.i25.3183

[5] Molaoa SZ. Prevalence of *Helicobacter pylori* infection and the incidence of the associated malignant and peptic ulcer disease (PUD) at Nelson Mandela Academic Hospital: A retrospective analysis. Journal of Drug Assessment. 2021;**10**(1):57-61. DOI: 10.1080/21556660.2020.1854560

[6] Awuku YA, Simpong DL, Alhassan IK, et al. Prevalence of *Helicobacter pylori* infection among children living in a rural setting in Sub-Saharan Africa. BMC Public Health. 2017;**17**:360. DOI: 10.1186/ s12889-017-4274-z

[7] Aitala P, Mutyaba M, Okeny S, Kasule NM, Kasule R, Ssedyabane F, et al. Prevalence and risk factors of *Helicobacter pylori* infection among children aged 1-15 years at Holy Innocents Children Hospital, Mbaraba, South Western Uganda. Journal of Tropical Medicine. 2019;**2019**:6. Article ID 9303072. DOI: 10.1155/ 2019/9303072

[8] Marks LJ. History of *H. Pylori*: What we do and don't know. 2018. Available from: http://www.everydayhealth. com/h-pylori/history-what-we-dont-know/. [Accessed: 2022-08-16]

[9] Mesquita MP, Jorge TM, Mantese AS, Filho DA, Berbert V, Rodrigues JJ. Relationship of *Helicobacter pylori* seroprevalence with the occurrence and severity of psoriasis. Anais Brasileiros de Dermatologia. 2017;**52**:92(1). DOI: 10.1590/ abd1806-4841.20174880

[10] Samily AM, Morshed MA. An update of laboratory diagnosis of *Helicobacter pylori* in the Kingdom of Saudi Arabia. Journal of Infection in Developing Countries. 2015;**9**(8):806-814. DOI: 10.355/jidc.542

[11] Lamont JT. Bacteriology and Epidemiology of *Helicobacter Pylori* Infection. In: Post TW, editor. UpToDate. Waltham, MA: UpToDate Inc. Available from: https://www.uptodate. com/contents/bacteriology-and-epidemiology-of-helicobacter-pylori-infection. [Accessed: August 14, 2022]

[12] Rojas B, Alonso M. Microbiological conditions for culturing *Helicobacter Pylori*. Revista colombiana de Gastroenterología. 2013;**28**(2): 94-99. Available from: http:// www.scielo.org.co/scielo. php?script=sci_arttext&pid=S0120-99572013000200002&lng=en

[13] Roesler BM. Introductory chapter: *Helicobacter pylori* - An overview of an old human microorganism. In: Roesler BM, editor. *Helicobacter Pylori* - New Approaches of an Old Human Microorganism. London: IntechOpen; 2019. Available from: https://www.intechopen.com/chapters/68813. DOI: 10.5772/intechopen.88806

[14] Andersen PL, Rasmussen L. *Helicobacter pylori*-coccoid forms, and biofilm formation. FEMS Immunology & Medical Microbiology. 2009;**56**(2):112-115. DOI: 10.1111/j.1574-695X.2009.00556.x

[15] Ansari S, Yamaoka Y. Current understanding and management of *Helicobacter pylori* infection: An updated appraisal. Version 1. F1000Research. 2018;7:F1000. Faculty Rev-721. DOI: 10.12688/f1000research.14149.1

[16] Kyle AB, Steensma PD, Shampo AM. Barry James Marshall-discovery of *Helicobacter pylori* as a cause of peptic ulcer. Stamp Vignette on Medical Science. 2016;**91**(5):E67-E68. DOI: 10.1016/j.May 06.2016.01.025

[17] Momtaz H, Dabiri H, Sound N, et al. Study of *Helicobacter pylori* genotype status in cows, sheep, goats, and human beings. BMC Gastroenterology. 2014;**14**:61. DOI: 10.1186/1471-230X-14-61

[18] Tsang T, Shrestha MP. *Helicobacter pylori* infection in peptic ulcer disease. In: Chai J, editor. Peptic Ulcer Disease. London: IntechOpen; 2011. Available from: https://www.intechopen.com/chapters/22941. DOI: 10.5772/24889

[19] Sarasota A, Prachasilchai W. The role of *Helicobacter spp.* Infection in domestic animals. In: Mozsik G, editor. Current Topics in Gastritis - 2012. London: IntechOpen; 2013. Available from: https://www.intechopen.com/chapters/41546. DOI: 10.5772/53054

[20] Okuda M, Lin Y, Kikuchi S. *Helicobacter pylori* infection in children and adolescents. Advanced in Experimental Medicine and Biology. 2019;**1149**:107-120. DOI: 10.1007/5584_2019_361. PMID: 31037557

[21] Korotkaya Y, Shores D. *Helicobacter pylori* in pediatric patients. Journal of American Academy of Pediatrics, Pediatrics in Review. 2020;**41**(11):585-592. DOI: 10.1542/pir.2019-0048

[22] Kayali S, Manfredi M, Gaiani F, Bianchi L, Bizzarri B, Leandro G, et al. *Helicobacter pylori*, transmission routes and recurrence of infection: State of the art. Acta Bio-Medica. 2018;**89**(8-S):72-76. DOI: 10.23750/abm.v89i8-S.7947

[23] Dawood K, Mamdooh I. Pathophysiology of *H. pylori*. In: Neri V, Ahmed M, editors. Esophagitis and Gastritis - Recent Updates. London: IntechOpen; 2021. Available from: https://www.intechopen.com/chapters/76213. DOI: 10.5772/intechopen.96763

[24] Kusters JG, van Vliet AH, Kuipers EJ. Pathogenesis of *Helicobacter pylori* infection. Clinical Microbiology Reviews. 2006;**19**(3):449-490. DOI: 10.1128/CMR.00054-05

[25] McGee J, Mobley LT. Pathogenesis of *Helicobacter pylori* infection. Current Opinion in Gastroenterology. 2000;**16**(1):24-31

[26] Cheng-Yen K, Bor-Shyang S, Jiunn-Jong W. *Helicobacter pylori* infection: An overview of bacterial virulence factors and pathogenesis. Biomedical Journal. 2016;**39**(1):14-23. ISSN 2319-4170. DOI: 10.1016/j.bj.2015.06.002

[27] Kao CY, Sheu BS, Wu JJ. *Helicobacter pylori* infection: An overview of bacterial virulence factors and pathogenesis. Biomedical Journal. 2016;**39**(1):14-23, ISSN 2319-4170. Available from: https://www.sciencedirect.com/science/article/pii/S2319417016000160

[28] Senbanjo OI, Oshikoya AK, Njokanma FO. *Helicobacter pylori* associated with breastfeeding, nutritional status, and recurrent abdominal pain in healthy Nigerian children. Journal of Infection in Developing Countries. 2014;**8**(4):448-453. DOI: 10.3855/JIDE.3196

[29] Abbas M, Sharif AF, Osman MS, Osman AM, El Sanousi SM, Magzoub M, et al. Prevalence and associated symptoms of *Helicobacter pylori* infection among schoolchildren in kassala state, East of Sudan. Interdisciplinary Perspectives on Infectious Diseases. 2018;**2018**. Article ID 4325752:5. DOI: 10.1155/2018/4325752

[30] Cochran JW. Peptic ulcer in children. MSD Manual Consumer Version. Available from: https://www.msdmanuals.com/home/children-s-health-issues/digestive-disorders-in-children/peptic-ulcer-in-children. Accessed on 14/08/2022

[31] Lamont JT. *Helicobacter pylori*. Gastroenterology at nemours children's health. Available from: https://kidshealth.org/en/parents/h-pylori.html. Accessed on 14/08/2022

[32] Ali AM, Elkhabit WF. Potential complication of *Helicobacter pylori* infection in children of non-urban community. Archives of Pediatric Infectious Diseases. 2015;**3**(2):e23512. DOI: 10.5812/pedinfect.23510

[33] Gulcan M, Ozen A, Karate OH, Vitrine A. Impact of *Helicobacter pylori* on growth: Is the infection or the mucosal disease related to growth impairment? Digestive Diseases and Sciences. 2010;**55**:2878-2886. DOI: 10.1007/S10620-009-1091-Y

[34] Silva CS, da Silva Júnior RT, de Sá Santos LK, Apolonio JS, da Costa BT, Cuzzuol BR, et al. Extragastric manifestations of *Helicobacter pylori* infection: A Commentary. Archives of Gastroenterology Research. 2021;**2**(3):102-109

[35] Tsay FW, Hsu PI. *H. pylori* infection and extra-gastroduodenal diseases. Journal of Biomedical Science. 2018;**25**:65. DOI: 10.1186/s12929-018-0469-6

[36] Tori R. What are the extragastric manifestations of *H. pylori* infection? Gastroenterology advisor. April 22, 2022. Available from: https://www.gastroenterologyadvisor.com/h-pylori-infection/what-are-the-extragastric-manifestations-of-h-pylori-infection/. Accessed on 18/08/2022

[37] Gravina AG, Priadko K, Ciamarra P, Granata L, Facchiano A, Miranda A, et al. Extra-gastric manifestations of *Helicobacter pylori* Infection. Journal of Clinical Medicine. 2020;**9**(12):3887. DOI: 10.3390/jcm9123887

[38] Wang YK, Kuo FC, Liu CJ, Wu MC, Shih HY, Wang SS, et al. Diagnosis of *Helicobacter pylori* infection: Current options and developments. World Journal of Gastroenterology. 2015;**21**(40):11221-11235. DOI: 10.3748/wjg.v21.i40.11221

[39] Salles N. *Helicobacter pylori* infection in elderly patients. In: Chai J, editor. Peptic Ulcer Disease. London: IntechOpen; 2011. DOI: 10.5772/23228. Available from: https://www.intechopen.com/chapters/22952

[40] Mounsey A, Leonard EA. Noninvasive diagnostic tests for *Helicobacter pylori* infection. American Family Physician. 2019;**100**(1):16-17. Available from: https://www.aafp.org/pubs/afp/issues/2019/0701/p16.html. Accessed on 14/08/2022

[41] Jemilohun CA, Otegbayo JA. *Helicobacter pylori* infection: Past, present, and future. Original article. 2016. Volume 23, Article 216, 22 Apr. 10.1164. pamj. 23.216.8852. Available from: https://www.panafrican-med-journal.com/content/article/23/216/full

[42] Santacroce L. *Helicobacter pylori* infection treatment & management. Medscape. Updated: July 21, 2021. Available from: https://emedicine.medscape.com/article/176938-treatment. Accessed on 14/08/2022

[43] Abadi ATB. Strategies used by *Helicobacter pylori* to establish persistence infection. World Journal of Gastroenterology. 2017;**23**(16):2870-2882. DOI: 10.3748/wjg.v23.i16.2870

[44] Chew CA, Lye TF, Ang D, Ang TL. The diagnosis and management of *H. pylori* infection in Singapore. Singapore Medical Journal. 2017;**58**(5):234-240. DOI: 10.11622/smedj.2017037

[45] Myran L, Zarbock DS. Management of *Helicobacter pylori* infection. US Pharm. Gastroenterology. 2018;**43**(4):27-32. Available from: https://www.uspharmacist.com/article/management-of-helicobacter-pylori-infection. Accessed on 19/08/2022

[46] Jung HK, Kang SJ, Lee YC, Yang HJ, Park SY, Shin CM, et al. Korean college of *Helicobacter* and upper gastrointestinal research. Evidence-based guidelines for the treatment of *Helicobacter pylori* infection in Korea 2020. Gut Liver. 2021;**15**(2):168-195. DOI: 10.5009/gnl20288

[47] Nester O, Johnsen KM, Sorbye SW, Halvorsen FA, Tonnessen T, Paulsen EJ, et al. *Helicobacter pylori* infected patients 15 years after successful eradication. PLoS ONE. 2020;**15**(9):e0238944. DOI: 10.1371/journal.pone.0238944

[48] Diaconu S, Predesco A, Moldoveanu A, Pop CS, Fierbinteanu-Braticevici C. *Helicobacter pylori* infection: Old and new. Journal of Medicine and Life. 2017;**10**(20):112-117. Available from: https://www.ncbi.nlm.nih.gov/pmc/articles/PMC5467250/#_Hn_sectitle

[49] Kouitcheu Mabeku LB, Eyoum BB, Tepap ZC, Tali Nguefack LD, Leundji H. Broad spectrum resistance in *Helicobacter pylori* isolated from gastric biopsies of patients with dyspepsia in Cameroon and efflux-mediated multi-resistance detection in MDR isolates. BMC Infectious Diseases. 2019;**19**:880. DOI: 10.1186/s12879-019-4536-8

[50] Parisi R, Iskandar IYK, Kontopantelis E, Augustin M, Griffiths CEM, Ashcroft DM, et al. National, regional, and worldwide epidemiology of psoriasis: A systematic analysis and modeling study. British Medical Journal. 2020;**369**:m1590. DOI: 10.1136/bmj.m1590

[51] Ashton WD. The psoriasis and psoriatic arthritis alliance - A positive approach; effective management. 2021. Available from: https://www.papaa.org/learn-about-psoriasis-and-psoriatic-arthritis/common-questions/the-history-of-psoriasis/part-one-the-history-of-psoriasis/. Accessed on 20/08/2022

[52] Rendon A, Schäkel K. Psoriasis pathogenesis and treatment. International Journal of Molecular Sciences. 2019;**20**(6):1475. DOI: 10.3390/ijms20061475

[53] Bu J, Ding R, Zhou L, Chen X, Shen E. Epidemiology of psoriasis and comorbid diseases: A narrative review. Frontiers in Immunology. 2022;**13**:880201. DOI: 10.3389/fimmu.2022.880201

[54] Armstrong AW, Mehta MD, Schupp CW, Gondo GC, Bell SJ, Griffiths CEM. Psoriasis prevalence in adults in the United States. JAMA Dermatology. 2021;**157**(8):940-946. DOI: 10.1001/jamadermatol.2021.2007

[55] Hein D. Psoriasis risk factors. Healthline. August 16, 2018. Available from: https://www.healthline.com/health/psoriasis/risk-factors. [Accessed: 2022/08/21]

[56] Kim WB, Jerome D, Yeung J. Diagnosis and management of psoriasis. Canadian Family Physician. 2017;**63**(4):278-285

[57] Langone NYU. Psoriasis. 2022. Available from: https://nyulangone.org/conditions/psoriasis/diagnosis. [Accessed: 2022/08/21]

[58] Michalek IM, Loring B. Global Report on Psoriasis. World Health Organization. 2016. pp. 1-35. Available from: https://apps.who.int/iris/bitstream/handle/10665/204417/9789241565189_eng.pdf.psoriasis?sequence=1. Accessed on 20/08/2022

[59] Onsun N, Arda Ulusal H, Su O, Beycan I, Biyik Ozkaya D, Senocak M. Impact of *Helicobacter pylori* infection on the severity of psoriasis and response to treatment. European Journal of Dermatology. 2012;**22**(1):117-120. DOI: 10.1684/ejd.2011.1579

[60] Marae AH, Shehata WA, Azmy R, Abousaeida AM. *Helicobacter pylori* infection in the palm and sole of psoriatic patients. Menoufia Medical Journal 2021;34:71-75. Available from: http://www.mmj.eg.net/text.asp?2021/34/1/71/312031

[61] Fathy G, Said M, Abdel-Raheem SM, Sanad H. *Helicobacter pylori* infection: A possible predisposing factor in chronic plaque-type psoriasis. Journal of The Egyptian Women's Dermatologic Society. 2010;7:39-43

[62] Cinar SL, Kartal D, Gur G, Borlu M, Alli N. The effect of *Helicobacter pylori* eradication on psoriasis course. Open Access Text. Global Dermatology. 2017;**4**(3):1-4. ISSN: 2056-7863. DOI: 10.15761/GOD.1000218

[63] Azizzadeh M, Nejad VZ, Ghorbani R, Pahlevan D. Relationship between *Helicobacter pylori* infection and psoriasis. Annals of Saudi Medicine. 2014;**34**(3):241-244. DOI: 10.5144/0256-4947.2014.241

[64] Meng-Che W, Sheng-Kai MK, Huang-Hsi C, Jing-Yang H, Cheng-Chung WJ. Relationship between *Helicobacter pylori* infection and psoriasis: A nationwide population-based longitudinal cohort study. Medicine. 2020;**99**(24):e20632. DOI: 10.1097/MD.0000000000020632